Contact Lenses in
Ophthalmology

Other 'Colour Manuals
in Ophthalmology'

Retinal Detachment
The Eye in Systemic Disease
Uveitis
all by Jack J Kanski

Contact Lenses in Ophthalmology

Michael S. Wilson, MB, BS, DO
Director of Contact Lens Services and
Associate Specialist in Ophthalmology,
Western Ophthalmic Hospital, London

Elisabeth A.W. Millis, MB, BS, DO
Deputy Director of Contact Lens Services and
Associate Specialist in Ophthalmology,
Western Ophthalmic Hospital, London

Butterworths
London   Boston   Singapore
Sydney   Toronto   Wellington

First published 1988

© **Butterworth & Co. (Publishers) Ltd, 1988**

British Library Cataloguing in Publication Data

Wilson, Michael S.
  Contact lenses in ophthalmology.
  1. Contact lenses
  I.Title   II. Millis, Elisabeth A.W.
  III. Series
  617.7'523

  ISBN 0–407–01440–3

Library of Congress Cataloging-in-Publication Data

Wilson, Michael S.
  Contact lenses in ophthalmology.

  Bibliography: p.
  Includes index.
  1. Contact lenses. I. Millis, Elisabeth A.W.
  II. Title.
  RE977.C6W55   1988   617.7'523   88-7372
  ISBN 0–407–01440–3

Laserset by Scribe Design, Gillingham, Kent
Printed by Toppan Printing Company (H.K.) Ltd, Hong Kong

Preface

This book has been written from the medical point of view. It is designed for those ophthalmologists who wish to start a contact lens practice, either in hospital or privately. It is also for those ophthalmologists who are seeing an increasing number of patients with contact lens-related problems both in hospital and private practice. We also hope it will be of help to optometrists, and others involved in contact lens practice, with regard to the medical problems which may occur.

We wish to thank Jack Kanski who suggested that the book be written, and Ron Marsh for his enthusiastic support. In the USA we would like to thank our colleagues Oliver Dabezies Jnr and Linsy Farris for their advice on the American aspect and, in particular, Jim Atwood for his immediate response to any queries. We would specially like to thank Peter Wright for reading Chapter 14 and the last half of Chapter 8, and for his very constructive comments.

The majority of the photographs have been taken by one of us (MSW) over the past 25 years. We wish to thank Sue Ford, the photographer at the Western Ophthalmic Hospital, for her professional help and advice. Many thanks are also due to Georgette Behar and Jane Grace for the hard work they have done in typing and word processing the manuscript.

The contact lens field is constantly changing due to takeovers of manufacturers, alterations in terminology, and innovations, which has meant constant alterations to the text. We would like to thank all the manufacturers for their time and patience in dealing with our queries.

Michael S. Wilson
Elisabeth Millis

Contents

List of abbreviations

AEC	Axial edge clearance		EW	Extended wear
AEL	Axial edge lift		FOZR	Front optic zone radius
BOZD	Back optic zone diameter		FVP	Front vertex power
BOZR	Back optic zone radius		HVID	Horizontal visible iris diameter
BPOD	Back peripheral optic diameter		HWC	High water content (60% and above)
BPOR	Back peripheral optic radius		K	Keratometer
BUT	Break up time (tear film)		LWC	Low water content (below 60%)
BVP	Back vertex power		pHEMA	Polyhydroxyethylmethacrylate
CAB	Cellulose acetate butyrate		PMMA	Polymethylmethacrylate
CL	Contact lens		PVA	Poly vinyl alcohol
CT	Centre thickness		PVP	Poly vinyl pyrrolidone
DC	Dioptre cylinder		RFO	Reduced front optic
Dk	Oxygen permeability		RGP	Rigid gas permeable
Dk/t	Oxygen transmissibility		SCL	Soft contact lens = Hydrogel = Hydrophilic
DS	Dioptre sphere			
DW	Daily wear		TD	Total diameter
EOP	Equivalent oxygen permeability		WW	Weekly wear
ET	Edge thickness			

1

History, indications and terminology of contact lenses

History of contact lenses

The idea of a contact lens was first considered by Herschel in 1823 who thought they were potentially useful in cases of corneal irregularity. It was for these patients and those with high astigmatism that contact lenses were first developed.

The earliest practical contact lenses were designed by Fick in 1888 and were scleral lenses. At the same time Kalt in Paris and Muller, in Germany, described the use of similar lenses to flatten the cornea in cases of keratoconus.

In 1932 Dallos, who was the originator of the modern impression method for fitting scleral lenses, improved the moulding technique and suggested the minimal clearance method for fitting the lenses. Further improvement in tear film exchange was gained when, in 1943, Bier fenestrated these lenses. The use of lighter, plastic, scleral lenses, was pioneered by Feinbloom, and Muller and Obrig in the late thirties. The material, polymethylmethacrylate (PMMA), which was much lighter than glass and easier to work, made possible the corneal lenses designed by Tuohy in 1948. The 1950s saw several workers throughout Europe and America experimenting with smaller, thinner lenses to improve tear fluid exchange and wearing time.

The problems associated with PMMA lens wear ensured that the search continued for alternative materials which would transmit more oxygen to the cornea and be more comfortable to wear. In 1960 Wichterle and Lim reported on the possible use of a hydrophilic plastic polymer, polyhydroxyethylmethacrylate (pHEMA), as a contact lens material and produced soft, spuncast lenses (Dreifus, 1978). The material had to be purified to improve the colour and further technical refinements were made before soft lenses became a clinical entity. The first lenses, in the USA, were the Hydron lenses by Bausch and Lomb (1966) which were spuncast and these were followed by the Griffin Bionite lenses (1967) which were lathe cut. Since then other co-polymers have been used with a view to further improving oxygen transmission by reducing lens thickness or increasing the water content of the material.

The most recent development has been the production of rigid gas-permeable (RGP) materials suitable for use as contact lenses. Cellulose acetatebutyrate (CAB) lenses became available in 1974 and since then lenses made from silicone resin, and silicone rubber, silicone/acrylate co-polymers, styrene and fluoro/silicone/acrylate materials have all been used. All aim to give improved oxygen transmission with reasonable wetting properties.

Advantages and disadvantages of contact lenses

The advantages of contact lenses

If a patient wishes to wear contact lenses there is usually a suitable lens available and compared to spectacles contact lenses provide:

1. A wider visual field.
2. Nearer to normal image size, particularly with lenses of 8.0 DS and over.
3. If anisometropia of 3.0 DS or more produces symptoms, the aneisokonia can usually be

1

reduced enough with contact lenses to allow fusion of the images.

4. Rigid lenses can improve the vision of an irregular cornea by the liquid (tear) lens between the cornea and the back surface of the contact lens. They can be used for keratoconus or corneal injury and after keratoplasty and refractive corneal surgery.
5. Rigid and soft bifocal lenses are available (Chapter 10) and the materials and their methods of manufacture are improving all the time.
6. Improved appearance.

Disadvantages of contact lenses

1. Low myopes may miss the base-in prism effect which they get with spectacles and there may be initial problems with close work. However the majority of patients can adjust to this in a short time.
2. Prisms to correct horizontal diplopia can only be incorporated in rigid scleral lenses. A base-down prism of up to three dioptres can be incorporated into a rigid corneal or soft contact lens, but the weight may cause the lens to drop.
3. Lenses must be inserted and removed daily in the majority of cases and carefully cleaned and disinfected after each wearing.
4. Lenses are easily lost and are more difficult to handle than spectacles.
5. Lenses are more expensive than spectacles to buy and to maintain.
6. Damage to the eye can occur from insertion and removal of contact lenses.
7. Infections are more common, particularly with extended wear soft lenses.
8. The quality of vision with soft lenses may not be as good as with spectacles or rigid contact lenses.
9. Rigid lenses do not protect against dust and other foreign bodies.
10. There is still a need for spectacles, when contact lenses are not worn.

Indications for contact lenses

Contact lenses are an alternative to glasses for anyone who has to wear glasses all the time, so long as there are no contra-indications.

Low refractive errors

Most of these patients prefer their appearance with contact lenses rather than with spectacles.

High refractive errors

High myopes benefit from the increase in image size obtained with contact lenses and this may be the only way of obtaining good vision in severe cases. A patient wearing $-23.0\,\mathrm{DS}$ in spectacles may have a visual acuity of 6/36 (180/20) with glasses, but 6/6 (20/20) with contact lenses and with an improved visual field.

Aphakic patients benefit from the reduction in the peripheral distortion, the magnification of image size, and absence of ring scotoma. This gives a greatly improved visual field and cosmetic appearance when contact lenses replace heavy spectacle lenses.

Anisometropia

Contact lenses are particularly useful to correct anisometropia greater than 4.0 DS. Obvious examples are unilateral aphakia and high myopia, when binocular vision may only be obtained by a contact lens.

Astigmatism

Irregular astigmatism is found in keratoconus, postkeratoplasty and associated with injured and scarred corneas. When spectacles do not provide adequate vision contact lenses are often successful and surgery may be avoided or postponed.

Occupational and environmental conditions

Occupations may affect the need and ability to wear contact lenses. Spectacles may be inappropriate for those in the performing arts. Surgeons using microscopes find contact lenses easier to wear than glasses. Dentists, who wear contact lenses, should wear protective spectacles over their lenses to protect their eyes and their contact lenses. This also applied to other lens wearers who are normally required to wear safety glasses at work. Cabin crews find that the low humidity of modern aircraft can make lens wear uncomfortable and large, soft lenses are preferable in dusty atmospheres, as particles are less likely to get

underneath them. In atmospheres with chemical, smoke and cooking fumes soft lenses can absorb the fumes from the air and a toxic keratitis may result.

Lenses for sport

The wider visual field is an advantage in many sports. It is important that the lenses remain centred with sudden eye movements and the larger, more stable, soft lenses are preferred, particularly for contact sports.

Therapeutic lenses

Large, high water, or very thin lower water content, soft lenses are used and are usually afocal. They can be used to treat corneal conditions such as bullous keratopathy and recurrent erosions (see Chapter 14).

Miscellaneous uses

Occasionally patients cannot wear spectacles because they have deformed or absent ears, allergies to spectacle frames, or trigemminal neuralgia associated with wearing glasses.

Factors influencing contact lens wear

Serious infected corneal ulcers may occur unnoticed by the patient particularly if a contact lens is worn on an anaesthetic cornea. Such ulcers are most likely to occur with extended wear lenses. However other conditions may influence the advisability of wearing a particular type of lens or any lens at all.

Systemic conditions

Skin disease

Acne rosacea may be exacerbated because the lens acts as an irritant causing vasodilatation of the face and conjunctiva. Psoriasis and neurodermatitis cause inflamed lids and irritation as skin cells are shed (Stein and Slatt, 1984).

Systemic drugs

Dry eyes may occur with atropine, hexamethonium, practolol, propranolol, systemic timolol, chlorpromazine and diazepam and similar substances (Frais and Bayley, 1979; Garston, 1986). Isotretinoin, which is used in the treatment of severe acne, may cause increased meibomian secretion and contact lens intolerance and bromhexine may increase lacrimal secretion (Manthorpe *et al.*, 1981 and Norn, 1985). Contraceptive pills are associated with dry eyes which can cause a reduced wearing time. Some women do find contact lens wear difficult during pregnancy and it may be preferable to delay fitting a new patient or new lenses until after delivery. Sulphasalazine (Riley, Flegg and Mandal, 1986) and rifampicin (Harris and Jenkins, 1985) have been found to discolour soft contact lenses.

Atopy

Atopic eczema, asthma and hay fever can cause ocular hyperaemia and epiphora so that lens wear may be difficult. They may also be associated with allergies to preservatives in the care solutions or a papillary response of the upper tarsal conjunctiva.

Hormonal disorders

In thyroid disease large soft lenses are usually better when there is lid retraction. Tear film abnormalities and altered corneal hydration are common during pregnancy, menstruation and menopause.

Handling problems

The commonest cause of difficulty handling lenses, which can occur at any age, is a psychological barrier to touching the eyes, producing lid spasm, epiphora and hand tremor. With increasing age joint deformities, intention tremor and loss of finger sensitivity, may occur.

Loss of one or more fingers or psoriasis of the skin or nails may also cause problems.

Local disease

Lids

Any active lid disease such as blepharitis, meibomitis, chalazion or stye should be treated before contact lenses are prescribed. In contact lens wearers a papillary response may cause itching and increased mucus secretion. However many teenagers have a papillary response prior to starting lens wear, and it is essential that the upper tarsal conjunctiva is examined before lenses are worn. An abnormal blink rate or distorted lid may reduce contact lens tolerance, because the eye becomes dry or the lid margin is irritated by the lens edge.

Corneal and conjunctival disease

Except where therapeutic soft lenses are indicated all active disease should be treated prior to commencing contact lens wear. This includes bacterial and viral keratitis and conjunctivitis, corneal ulcers and allergic reactions.

Tear film

Reduced or abnormal tear film will increase the adaptation period, decrease wearing time, cause discomfort and reduce vision. Problems will be aggravated with soft lenses as fluid evaporates from the anterior surface and is replaced by tear fluid. A lens which becomes dry will shrink and tighten to indent the conjunctiva with its edge. Tight fitting rigid lenses may not permit adequate tear exchange beneath the lens because lens movement is markedly reduced.

Mucin deficiency is due to conjunctival goblet cell destruction by diseases such as pemphigoid, Stevens–Johnson syndrome, burns and trachoma.

The aqueous secretion of the tear film is affected by disorders of the lacrimal gland and the accessory lacrimal glands. Kerato-conjunctivitis sicca, Sjogrens disease, conjunctival burns and lacrimal gland surgery may all result in an abnormal or reduced aqueous secretion.

The lipid layer is rarely affected but meibomitis may alter its constituents. In a marginally dry eye a thin soft lens, or a high water content soft lens may be used, provided the patient instills copious N-saline drops. A rigid lens is preferred for definitely dry eyes.

Topical drugs

Topical eye drops such as neutral adrenaline (epinephrine) will stain soft lenses yellow and brown. The preservatives in many contact lens solutions and eye drops, notably benzalkonium chloride (BKC) which is toxic to the cornea, can bind to lenses causing irritation, and sensitivity reactions may occur, particularly with thiomersal (D'Arcy, 1986).

Surgical complications

Thin drainage blebs if damaged may result in endophthalmitis, therefore the size and type of lens should be chosen to avoid trauma. A loose suture can act as a wick for intraocular infection and if deeply placed it should be removed before starting lens wear.

Motivation

This is the most important single factor in successful lens wear, particularly with children. They should be keen to wear lenses, and not just to please their parents. Some patients are psychologically unsuited to contact lenses and may concoct a variety of reasons why they have not managed to wear them.

Financial

The cost of supplying, fitting, and maintaining lenses together with the cost of follow-up appointments must be discussed with the patient so that they understand that there is a continuous commitment.

Contact lens terminology

There are many terminologies for the different types of contact lens. Originally there were only scleral lenses, then PMMA lenses. Hydrogel or hydrophilic lenses were subsequently called soft or flexible lenses. Gas permeable hard lenses have tended to be called rigid lenses and some authorities have used the terms rigid and flexible to cover all lenses. We have adopted the terminology of:

1. Polymethylmethacrylate (PMMA) scleral lenses which extend over the cornea onto the conjunctiva overlying the sclera.
2. PMMA corneal lenses. These lenses are smaller than the overall diameter of the cornea.
3. Rigid gas-permeable corneal lenses (RGP).
4. Soft lenses which are hydrophilic and are larger than the cornea.

The general term 'rigid' lens is used to include both PMMA and RGP lenses. Lenses are worn to correct refractive errors (refractive lenses), as treatment for an ocular condition (therapeutic) or to disguise an unsightly eye (cosmetic). The term cosmetic is sometimes used to refer to lenses which correct low refractive errors, and these are included in the refractive group.

The terminology relevant to contact lenses is now discussed (Figure 1.1).

The Optic Zone (OZ) is the refractive area of the lens. It has an anterior surface, the front optic (FO) and a posterior surface the back optic (BO). The latter is the 'fitting curve' of the lens and is designed to conform to the shape of the eye. The OZ is described by the *Front and Back Optic Zone Diameters (FOZD and BOZD)* and their corresponding radii *(FOZR and BOZR)*.

The radius of curvature of the BOZR may be measured, by a keratometer, in millimetres or as the dioptric power of the cornea.

Back Peripheral Curves (BPCs) are flatter than the BOZR to conform to the flatter corneal periphery. There may be one or more BPCs, depending on the overall size of the lens. The larger the lens the more BPCs are possible. An OZ with a single PC constitutes a bi-curve (C2) lens. Tri-curve (C3) lenses are usually used for lenses greater than 9.0 mm diameter, and multi-curve lenses are possible. Continually flattening curves with no junctions can be made e.g. aspheric periphery. The construction of the BPCs in a tri-curve lens is shown in Figure 1.1. The overall diameter of the lens is the Total Diameter (TD). The BPCs simulate the corneal curvature, improve tear exchange if well designed and support the tear meniscus which centralizes the lens.

The junctions (J1, J2 etc) between two PCs should be blended, using a wax tool with a curve midway between the two, to aid tear exchange and reduce discomfort. Blends may be light, medium or heavy, depending on their width. Blended junctions are called transitions.

The centre thickness (CT) of a lens is measured at its geometric centre. A thin lens is usually more comfortable than a thick one, provided it is possible to make a good edge. Some gas-permeable materials are fragile, and the CT of a lens may need to be greater than for the equivalent PMMA lens to minimize breakages. Oxygen permeability is related to lens thickness (see Chapter

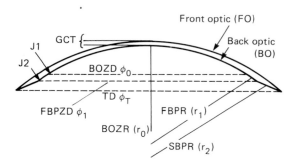

Figure 1.1 Diagram to show the design parameters for a tri-curve lens (GCT, geometric centre thickness; BOZD, back optic zone diameter; FBPZD, first back peripheral zone diameter; TD, total diameter; BOZR, back optic zone radius; FBPR, first back peripheral radius; SBPR, second back peripheral radius; J1, junction of optic zone and first back peripheral curve (FBPC); and J2, junction of the FBPC and the Second back peripheral curve (SBPC))

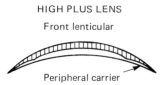

Figure 1.2 Reduced front optic to reduce the weight and centre thickness of a high plus lens

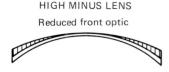

Figure 1.3 Lenticulating a high minus lens reduces the edge thickness of the lens

2) and care must be taken to avoid increasing thickness to the extent that oxygen permeability is detrimentally reduced. Single cut high plus lenses have thick centres but a lenticular form will reduce the CT (Figure 1.2). CT depends on the power, diameter and method of manufacture of the lens.

The radial edge thickness (ET) and shape of the lens edge is important for comfort. It is measured normal to the front surface of the lens at a specified distance from the edge and should be 0.08–0.12 mm thick, smooth and well-rounded. The edge thickness of a high minus lens can be reduced by a Reduced Front Optic (RFO) (Figure 1.3).

Lenses may be stabilized by prism ballast or truncation of the lens (see Chapter 10).

Rigid lenses can be made from tinted material to make them easier to locate, particularly on the eye. Soft lenses may be tinted for cosmetic reasons, to alter the colour of the iris. Tinted cosmetic lenses are also used to disguise unsightly eyes (see Chapter 13). The most common tint for a rigid lens is light grey, as this does not affect colour values.

The front curve of the lens determines the power and this is again determined by the BOZR.

References

D'ARCY, P.F. (1986) Drug interactions with soft contact lenses. *Pharmacy International*, September, 219–220

DREIFUS, M. (1978) The development of pHEMA for contact lens wear. In *Soft Lenses: Clinical and Applied Technology* (ed. M. Ruben), Ballière Tindall, London, pp. 7–16

FRAISE, M.A. and BAYLEY, T.J. (1979) Ocular reaction to Timolol Maleate. *Postgraduate Medical Journal*, **55**, 884–885

GARSTON, M. (1986) Untoward effects of pharmaceutical agents. *Contemporary Optometry*, **5**, 23–32

HARRIS, J. and JENKINS, P. (1985) Discolouration of soft contact lenses by rifampicin. *The Lancet*, November 16, 1133

MANTHORPE, R., FROST-LARSEN, K., ISAGER, H., et al. (1981) Lack of lacrimal gland improvement by Na-872 in Sjogrens syndrome. *Acta Ophthalmologica* (Copenhagen), **59**, 336–346

NORN, M. (1985) The effects of drugs on tear flow. *Transactions of the Ophthalmic Society of the United Kingdom*, **104**, 410–414

RILEY, S.A., FLEGG, P.T. and MANDAL, B.K. (1986) Contact lens staining due to sulphasalazine. *The Lancet*, April 26, 972

STEIN, H.A. and SLATT, B.J. (1984) *Fitting guide for rigid and soft contact lenses. A practical approach*, 2nd edn, C.V. Mosby Co., St Louis, Toronto, pp. 21–30

WICHTERLE, O. and LIM, L.W.F. (1960) Hydrophilic gels for biological uses. *Nature*, **185**, 117

Further reading

BIER, N. (1948) The practice of ventilated contact lenses. *Optician*, **116**, 497–501

DALLOS, J. (1936) Contact glasses, the invisible spectacles. *Archives of Opthalmology* (New York), **15**, 617–623

DALLOS, J. (1938) The individual fitting of contact glasses. *Transactions of the Ophthalmic Society of the United Kingdom*, **57**, 509–520

FEINBLOOM, W. (1937) A plastic contact lens. *American Journal of Optometry*, **14**, 41–49

FICK, A.E. (1888) A contact lens. (Translation by C.H. May) *Archives of Ophthalmology*, **19**, 215–226

HERSCHEL, J.F.W. (1845) 'Light', Section XII 'Of the structure of the eye and of vision.' *Encyclopaedia metropolitana*, **4**, 396–404

NISSEL, G. (1965) The Mullers of Wiesbaden. *Optician*, **150**, 591–594

OBRIG, T.E. (1937) Fitting of contact lenses for persons with ametropia. *Archives of Ophthalmology* (New York), **17**, 1089–1120

2

The anatomy, physiology and bacteriology of the eye related to contact lens wear

The back surface of a contact lens overlies part or all of the cornea. Rigid corneal contact lenses are smaller than the cornea, rigid scleral and soft semi-scleral lenses are larger than the cornea. The anterior surface of the lens is related to the upper and lower palpebral conjunctiva. Correct blinking (see below) produces a vertical and rotary movement of both corneal and soft lenses, unless they have been stabilized to prevent rotation (see Chapter 10). The eyelids spread the tear film evenly over the surface of the eye with each complete blink and also wipe the lens clean to maintain comfort and good vision. The important features of these structures in relation to contact lens wear are discussed in this chapter.

The cornea

The cornea is the most anterior structure of the eye and its main refracting surface.

Topography

The cornea is approximately elliptical with average vertical and horizontal diameters of 11.5 mm and 12 mm respectively. The central portion, the optic cap, is 5–7 mm in diameter and, normally, almost spherical. The cornea flattens towards the periphery and this must be taken into consideration when designing a contact lens. The cornea is thinner centrally (0.50 mm) than peripherally

(0.75 mm). It is 5/6 adult size at birth when the average radius of curvature is 7.00 mm and this increases to an average of 8.00 mm by six years.

Anatomy

Epithelium

This comprises 5–6 layers of cells, the superficial layers of which have tight junctions. The cells of the deeper layers are closely bound together with desmosomes whilst the middle layer wing cells interdigitate closely with one another and have narrow intercellular spaces. As a result the epithelium forms a barrier between the tear film and the deeper corneal structures.

All superficial cells bear microvilli and microplicae which increase in size as they near the surface, where they stabilize the mucin content of the tear film.

Changes occurring in the epithelium associated with contact lens wear

1. Hard lenses can reduce the microvilli and alter cell shape (Hamano, 1978). They can also disrupt the tight junctions and dilate the intercellular spaces (Bergmanson and Chu, 1982), causing an increase in the permeability of the epithelium, and oedema may occur.
2. Soft lenses may result in thinning of the cornea due to cell loss (Bergmanson, Ruben and Chu, 1985).

7

3. Epithelial microcysts occur with all types of lens but are most commonly found with extended wear soft lenses. The cause is unknown (Humphreys, Larke and Parrish, 1980).
4. Preservatives in soft contact lens solutions can damage the epithelium by disrupting the intercellular spaces and reducing the microvilli (Brewitt and Feurerhake, 1980).
5. Changes also occur in the epithelium as a result of trauma or anoxia which can cause oedema and ulceration.

Stroma

The stroma consists of an orderly arrangement of collagen fibrils in a mucopolysaccharide matrix containing glucoseaminoglycans (GAGS). Contact lens wear usually results in some degree of stromal oedema, even though minimal. This causes separation of the collagen fibrils which may be sufficient to cause loss of transparency (Hart and Farrell, 1969).

Endothelium

The single layer of endothelial cells is firmly bound together with tight junctions, interdigitations and macula adherens which create a barrier preventing the entry of aqueous fluid into the stroma.

Three endothelial changes, visible with the specular microscope, occur in association with contact lens wear (Efron and Holden, 1986a and b). These are:

Blebs These small swellings, on the posterior endothelial surface, develop as soon as a contact lens is inserted. They reach a peak in 30 minutes and subside to a low level in an hour. With the specular microscope they appear as dark areas due to loss of specular reflection and vanish rapidly when the lens is removed.

Polymegathism The normal endothelial cell count is 2500–4000 cells per mm² in the young and approximately half that number in the elderly. Polymegathism is a variation in cell size which occurs with increasing age and, almost immediately, when any contact lens is worn. MacRae *et al*, (1986) found the changes induced by rigid lenses were greater with longer periods of wear and were not completely reversible.

Bedewing 'Droplets', which may be found in clusters on the posterior endothelial surface, are thought to be collections of inflammatory cells, possibly due to a mild anterior uveitis associated with contact lens wear. Bedewing causes discomfort resulting in a reduction in the wearing time which resolves rapidly once lens wear is stopped although bedewing may be visible for several months.

Corneal metabolism

Glucose

The main source of glucose for corneal metabolism is from the aqueous. Eighty five per cent of glucose is stored as glycogen in the epithelium, which is metabolized anaerobically via the Embden–Meyerhof pathway to produce lactate, the rest is metabolized aerobically (Holden *et al.*, 1987). During contact lens wear glycogen is mobilized and ATP levels fall (Thoft and Friend, 1975). The fall in glycogen levels appears to be related to hypoxia and trauma. If lactic acid levels rise corneal swelling and oedema may occur (Smelser and Chen, 1955).

Oxygen

Oxygen is obtained from the atmosphere via the tear film and, to a lesser extent, from the aqueous and the limbal blood vessels. When the eye is closed oxygen is supplied by the palpebral vessels. With the eye open the oxygen tension in the tears is 20.7 kPa (155 mmHg), but falls to 7.3 kPa (55 mmHg) with the eyes closed. The amount of oxygen necessary to prevent corneal oedema has been variously reported to be between 1.5% and 10% of the atmospheric oxygen pressure (Polse and Mandell, 1970; Mandell and Farrell, 1980; Holden, Sweeney and Sanderson, 1984). The variation in the findings reflects the different methods used to assess the problem.

All contact lenses affect corneal metabolism, depending on the type, thickness and fit of lens used. A large, scleral PMMA lens will tend to have the greatest effect, and a silicone rubber lens the least.

PMMA corneal lenses allow imperceptible oxygen transmission through the lens but atmos-

pheric oxygen readily dissolves in the tear film. Sufficient oxygen can only reach the cornea beneath the lens by means of the 'tear pump' resulting from movement of the lens on the cornea during blinking. As the eye closes the lens moves down on the cornea and tears are expressed from under the lens. As the eye opens the lens moves up and away from the cornea, creating a negative pressure under the lens which draws in more oxygenated tears, which is termed venting (Klyce, Farris and Dabezies, 1984). The effectiveness of the tear pump depends on the volume of tear fluid available and the amount which is exchanged with each blink. A reduced blink rate causes a decrease in oxygen supplies to the cornea.

Soft lenses transmit oxygen to the cornea via the water contained in the lens, the transmission being directly related to the water content of the lens material and its thickness. High water content lenses will transmit more oxygen than low water content lenses, and thinner lenses more than thick ones. With soft lenses there is minimal tear pump action.

RGP lenses can transmit oxygen not only through the lens, the supply being dependent on the lens material and its thickness, but also via the tear pump mechanism (see Chapter 3). It has been estimated (O'Neal, Polse and Sarver, 1984) that the minimum oxygen transmissability to prevent corneal oedema is 75×10^{-9} and this is equivalent to an oxygen tension of 5.3 kPa (40 mmHg). Clinically RGP lenses with a lower oxygen transmission are satisfactory in most cases of daily wear, because of the tear pump contribution to the oxygen supply. Hypoxia results in increased glucose utilization and lactate production, and may produce oedema. There is an increased risk of oedema when lenses are worn during sleep, as the already lowered oxygen tension will be reduced still further by the contact lens, and the tear pump effect will be minimal.

Hydration

The cornea consists of 78% water due to the high water-binding capacity of the stromal proteoglycans, and the overall result of osmotic forces acting on the cornea is to encourage water to enter the stroma. Failure to prevent too much fluid entering the cornea causes oedema with loss of transparency and reduced vision. *Corneal hydration*

is regulated by mechanisms situated in the epithelium and endothelium as follows:

1. Because of their structure these layers form physical barriers to the passage of fluid (see above).
2. Both layers contain cationic pumps which actively transport ions across the barriers with water following passively (Maurice, 1972). The major mechanism is situated in the endothelium and a bicarbonate pump is postulated (Hodson and Miller, 1976).

By these means the cornea is normally maintained in a state of relative dehydration. Failure of either of the barriers or of the pumps results in corneal oedema which can affect the stroma and/or the epithelium. In stromal oedema the fluid collects intercellularly, and results in corneal swelling under the area consistently covered by the lens. It is usually central with PMMA lenses, but affects the whole cornea with soft lenses. Epithelial oedema associated with contact lens wear, is characterized by intercellular fluid, cell shrinkage and loss of desmosomes. Similar changes are seen in association with hypotonic solutions, which suggest that lactate accumulates in the stroma when the lens is worn, and creates an osmotic gradient between the stroma and the epithelium (Holden and Swarbrick, 1987).

Epithelial oedema, in a PMMA lens wearer, is best observed with the slit-lamp using the sclerotic scatter technique. In a dark room a slit-lamp beam about 2 mm wide, is focused on the temporal limbus so that, with the eye looking straight ahead, the light is totally internally reflected by the cornea. The cornea is viewed without the microscope, from the nasal side, and an oedematous area will appear as a central, circular grey/white area. Stromal oedema is more diffuse and therefore difficult to see but causes increased corneal thickness which can be assessed by eye and measured with the pachometer. It may cause distortion of the keratometry mires and a steepening of the K-readings when the central cornea is affected.

Corneal sensation

Normal corneal sensation, which is essential for safe contact lens wear, should be assessed in all patients. In those wishing to wear contact lenses

as a cosmetic alternative to spectacles, reduced sensation is a contra-indication. However patients who need lenses for medical reasons, which includes aphakia, often have some reduction in sensation. They can be fitted with contact lenses providing they are kept under close supervision and adequate emergency facilities are available.

Corneal sensitivity tends to reduce with increasing age and also with contact lens wear, intra-ocular operations, fifth nerve palsy and diabetes. PMMA lenses cause a greater reduction in corneal sensitivity than soft lenses. Cessation of wear is followed by recovery of sensation. Corneal sensation may be measured quantitatively by the Cochet and Bonnet aesthesiometer or, clinically, by touching a wisp of cotton wool to the cornea and observing the reflex blink of the other eye.

Patients with reduced corneal sensation should understand that help must be sought urgently if the eye is red, even though the eye is not painful.

Corneal neovascularization

Limbal hyperaemia is a common feature of all types of contact lens wear and if persistent may lead to eventual corneal neovascularization (McMonnies, 1984) and must be kept under observation when it occurs. New vessels occur as a response by existing blood vessels to metabolic or vasoproliferative factors. Neovascularization is moderately common with scleral lenses especially when there is constriction of limbal vessels or chronic oedema. It is uncommon with PMMA lenses except when they override the limbus, or are worn for long periods, under dry eye conditions. It is most frequently seen with large, thick, soft, lenses especially when the fit is too tight (see Chapter 8).

Tear film

A normal tear film, with adequate venting under the lens, is essential for successful contact lens wear. When dry the corneal surface is no longer smooth and the visual acuity is reduced. The precorneal tear film transports gases to and from the cornea and contains bactericidal substances

(see below). Increased tear film from a watering eye washes away debris and foreign bodies.

The configuration of precorneal tear film between the cornea and a contact lens will vary depending on the lens–cornea relationship. Since the refractive indices of the lens, tears and cornea differ the tear fluid forms a refracting lens, and the power of this 'liquid lens' has to be considered when calculating the power of a contact lens. If a contact lens is fitted flatter than the mean keratometer reading, the liquid lens will add minus power to the contact lens, and if fitted steeper will add plus power.

Structure of tear film

Classically the tear film is regarded as having three layers, a semi-solid layer and two fluid layers.

1. Mucin is derived from the conjunctival goblet cells, the Crypts of Henle and the glands of Moritz, and forms a hydrophilic surface on the corneal epithelium which stabilizes the tear film.
2. The aequeous layer is formed by the lacrimal and the accessory lacrimal glands. It prevents the cornea drying and contains substances with antibacterial actions such as lysozyme, lactoferrin and β-lysin. Secretory IgA, IgG and IgM have also been found (Jordan and Baum, 1980).
3. The outermost, lipid layer, which is formed from the secretions of the meibomian glands and glands of Zeis and Moll, prevents evaporation of the underlying layers.

Conjunctival disease causing damage to the goblet cells results in mucin deficiency and altered wetting of the cornea whilst female hormonal changes, lacrimal surgery or conjunctival disease can reduce the aqueous layer. A lipid deficiency is rare, more often there is an alteration in the constituents of the meibomian secretion due to disease such as blepharitis (see below).

Examination of the tear film

The state of the tear film is important in assessing a patient's suitability for contact lenses, and should be examined in detail.

The amount of tear film meniscus above the lower eyelid can be assessed with the slit-lamp,

first without, and then with fluorescein. A minimal tear meniscus, particularly if it is associated with debris, suggests a tear deficiency.

The tear film break-up time (BUT) is measured by instilling a touch of fluorescein to the conjunctiva above the cornea and getting the patient to blink completely closed and then keep the eyes open. The time, in seconds, between the blink and the first appearance of a dry spot on the cornea is the BUT. The normal BUT is 30–60 seconds, a BUT of less than ten seconds suggests an abnormal tear film and a mucus deficiency (Lang and Hamill, 1973). It has recently been suggested that the BUT may be reduced by fluorescein (Holly, 1987).

Schirmers test measures the amount of fluid absorbed on to standard absorbent paper strips in five minutes. Values greater than 5.0 mm are normal.

Tear film and contact lenses

Normal tear film dynamics are radically altered when a contact lens is placed on the eye. Increased evaporation of tears occurs, and an increased volume of fluid is needed to keep the eye moist. A dry eye may result from a reduction in quantity or alteration in the quality of the tear film, and may cause irritation, discomfort and reduced wearing time of the lenses. Reduced tear volume produces an inadequate tear film meniscus, debris in the tear film and beneath the lens, a reduced lens movement, and increased deposit formation on the lenses (Farris, 1987). The treatment is the use of copious lubricating eye drops. The patient should be advised to avoid hot air from car heaters or hair dryers and to blink correctly and more frequently (see below).

Mucin abnormalities may cause punctate epithelial staining and strands of mucus to accumulate in the tear film. Acetylcysteine is useful as a mucolytic and lubricating drops, particularly those such as Liquifilm Tears (Allergan) and Sno-tears (Smith and Nephew Pharmaceuticals) which contain polyvinyl alcohol 1.4%, improve wetting. They are not suitable for use with soft lenses because they contain benzalkonium chloride as a preservative. Lipid abnormalities, due to chronic blepharitis with excessive meibomian secretion, can result in a coated lens and reduced visual

acuity. Warm compresses can help to soften the accumulation of secretion at the gland openings. Local daily antibiotic drops and ointments at night can be used effectively on the lid margins. Systemic tetracycline 250 mg b.d. for six weeks may be necessary for some patients. Greasy lenses should be cleaned with a surfactant cleaner such as Miraflow (Ciba Vision Contactasol). Staining corneal lesions due to localized drying, may occur at the three and nine o'clock peripheries as a result of altered blinking, with rigid corneal lenses (see Chapter 7).

The osmotic pressure of the tear film is equivalent to 0.9% NaCl (Aquavella, 1975). Soft contact lenses immersed in hypotonic solutions will swell, and in hypertonic solutions will shrink. This property has been used in some cleaning regimes where lens shrinkage helps to loosen debris from the lens surface. The lens must be soaked in an isotonic solution, before replacing them on the eye, to restore its size, curvature and power to normal.

The eyelids

Function of the lids

Correct blinking distributes the precorneal tear film over the whole corneal surface. As the lids close the lipid layer of the tear film is compressed between the lid margins, to become considerably thicker. As the lids open the lipid layer thins and is spread rapidly over the aqueous layer, as if it were attached to the lid margins, so that the aqueous layer is continuously covered. An irregular lid surface or lid margin can affect the even distribution of the tear film.

Correct blinking is essential for successful contact lens wear. The lids and the contact lens act together as a pump to exchange the precorneal tear film under the lens, and oxygenate the cornea, which is particularly important with rigid lenses. For correct blinking the patient should close their eyes completely, as though they were closing their eyes to sleep, and never squeeze closed, particularly with rigid lenses. Many people blink incompletely, which can be termed 'flick blinking', when the lids are half closed (Wilson, 1971).

Lens–lid relationship

A lens which is displaced on the eye may alter the contour of the corneal surface and the normal blink pattern, causing dry areas to occur. There may be increased awareness of the lens by the upper lid margin. This can be reduced by fitting thinner lenses which also allow the upper lid to wipe the affected area more completely as it does not 'bridge over' the adjacent corneal area. Improved blinking and artificial tear drops should also help. Interpalpebral lenses tend to produce increased upper lid margin lens awareness. A 'lid attachment' fitting lens has its upper margin beneath the upper lid, and moves with the upper lid as recommended by Korb and Korb for fitting PMMA lenses (see Chapter 7).

Contact lenses have been lost and have eventually been found, often after many months, encysted in the upper lid (Jones, Livesy and Wilkins, 1987). It is essential to doubly evert the upper lid in patients where there is a history of lens loss, or to sweep a fine glass rod under the upper lid (Chapters 7 and 8).

Bacteriology of contact lens wear

All contact lenses are potential sources of infection and the risk is increased with an unhealthy cornea, and a dry eye.

The most commonly reported pathogen is *Pseudomonas* (Kapetansky *et al.*, 1964; Hassman and Sugar, 1983; Galentine *et al.*, 1984) but *Staphylococcus aureus* and *epidermidis*, α-haemolytic *Streptococcus* and *Serratia marcescens* have all been found associated with lenses, carrying cases and care solutions. *Pseudomonas* has been shown to attach to hydrogel lenses in numbers which increase with time (Duran *et al.*, 1987). Soft contact lenses, and probably other types, act as substrates because they are covered with a polysaccharide biofilm which interacts with bacteria that adhere to the surface. A slime covered environment is formed for the bacteria and the lens acts as an inoculum for unhealthy corneal epithelium (Slusher *et al.*, 1987).

A recent report (Cremons *et al.*, 1987) suggests that applying a pad and bandage to contact lens wearers with apparent corneal abrasions, who subsequently developed *Pseudomonas* infection within twenty-four hours, was more likely to result in corneal scarring than in lens wearers with *Pseudomonas* infection in general. These patients developed severe pain whilst wearing the pad. All corneal ulcers should be regarded as infected until proved otherwise by bacteriological culture. Any patient who is padded, for a corneal abrasion, should be warned to return immediately if more pain develops. Treatment is commenced with intensive tobramycin eyedrops, while awaiting the swab report, as some strains of *Pseudomonas* are resistant to gentamicin. All patients should be seen daily until the ulcer has healed.

The ocular bacterial flora of contact lens wearers does not differ significantly from non-lens wearers and the source of infection is often the carrying case (Winkler and Dixon, 1964). Both wet and dry stored lenses showed a high incidence of bacterial contamination which may be due to the tear film evaporating on an improperly cleaned lens, causing protein which forms a good culture medium, to concentrate on the lens (Dixon, 1964). Corneal infection can also occur from poor lens hygiene and from the insertion of a contaminated lens by the clinician.

A wide variety of yeasts and fungi have been found contaminating contact lenses (Kapetansky *et al.*, 1964; Ormerod and Smith, 1986; Wilson and Ahearn, 1986). The fungal hyphae may penetrate the substance of soft lenses and reach the cornea. The growth occurs as a furry grey-brown patch on the lens (Figures 8.18, 8.19), and may produce punctate epithelial staining with fluorescein and stromal infiltrates. The patient may complain of irritation and blurred vision.

Acanthamoeba keratitis has been reported associated with contact lenses (Mannis *et al.*, 1986; Cohen *et al.*, 1987). The majority of cases have occurred in soft lens wearers using home-made saline but other lenses may also be involved if unsterile solutions are used (Koenig *et al.*, 1987). *Acanthamoeba* causes an intractable keratitis with severe pain and a stromal ring infiltrate occurs late in the disease. The diagnosis may be made by corneal biopsy and paracentesis (McClellan and Coster, 1987), and using immunofluorescent techniques or innoculation into Culbertson's medium. Recurrences have been reported even after corneal grafting. The condition should be suspected in a contact lens wearer who has painful stromal

infiltrates. Treatment is frequently unsatisfactory but propamidine isethionate 0.1% (Brolene) and neomycin should be tried initially (Easty, 1988).

AIDS and contact lenses

HIV virus has been isolated from tear fluid and, experimentally, from soft contact lenses (Tervo *et al.*, 1986). There is therefore a potential risk of infection from an HIV positive patient wearing contact lenses.

The disinfection of contact lens trial sets is of paramount importance. The virus is susceptible to 3% hydrogen peroxide solution, sodium hypochlorite, isopropyl alcohol and household bleach (DHSS report, 1986; Report of US Food and Drug Administration, 1986; Faculty of Ophthalmologists, 1986). Hydrogen peroxide 3% is available in the Contactasol 10:10 regime (Ciba Vision Contactasol), as Lensept in the Septicon system (Ciba Vision Contactasol) and as Oxysept 1 (Allergan) for use with contact lenses.

Innoculated, unworn lenses have been effectively disinfected using surfactant cleaners such as Boston cleaner, Pliagel, Miraflow and Softmate Cleaning has been shown to be particularly effective when followed by chemical or thermal disinfection (Vogt *et al.*, 1986).

Softabs (Alcon) are chlorine releasing tablets which the manufacturers claim are effective against the AIDS virus. It is recommended that trial lenses should be immersed in Softabs for four hours.

Aerotabs (Sauflon Pharmaceuticals) are similar and contain a halazone which releases chlorine.

The preferred method is to clean trial lenses with a surfactant cleaner and then disinfect in Softabs or Aerotabs which do not require neutralizing.

References

Anatomy

BERGMANSON, J. and CHU, L.W.F. (1982) Corneal response to rigid contact lens wear. *British Journal of Ophthalmology*, **66**, 667–675

BERGMANSON, J., RUBEN, M. and CHU, L.W.F. (1985) Epithelial morphological response to soft hydrogel contact lenses. *British Journal of Ophthalmology*, **69**, 373–379

BREWITT, H. and FEUERERHAKE, C. (1980) The effect of disinfecting systems for soft contact lenses on the corneal epithelium – a scanning electron microscope study. *The Contact Lens Journal*, **9**, 19–21

EFRON, N. and HOLDEN, B. (1986a) A review of some common contact lens complications. Part I: The corneal epithelium and stroma. *Optician*, **192**, August 1 21–26

EFRON, N. and HOLDEN, B. (1986b) A review of some common contact lens complications. Part 2: The corneal endothelium and conjunctiva. *Optician*, **192**, September 5, 17–21, 24 and 29

HAMANO, H. (1978) Fundamental research on the effects of contact lenses on the eye. In *Soft Contact Lenses; Clinical and Applied Technology* (ed. M. Ruben), Baillière Tindall, London, pp. 121–142

HART, R.W. and FARREL, R.A. (1969) Light scattering in the cornea. *Journal of the Optometric Society of America*, **59**, 766

HUMPHREYS, J.A., LARKE, J.R. and PARRISH, S.T. (1980) Microepithelial cysts observed in extended wear contact lens wearing subjects. *British Journal of Ophthalmology*, **64**, 888–889

MACRAE, S.M., MATSUDA, M., SHELLANS, S. *et al.* (1986) The effects of hard and soft contact lenses on the corneal endothelium. *American Journal of Ophthalmology*, **102**, 50–57

Physiology

AQUAVELLA, J. (1975) Corneal physiology and the contact lens. *Contact and Intraocular Lens Medical Journal*, **1**, 121–125

FARRIS LINSY, R. (1987) Contact lens wear in the management of the dry eye. *International Ophthalmology Clinics*, **27**, 54–60

HODSON, S. and MILLER, F. (1976) The bicarbonate ion pump in the endothelium which regulates the hydration of the rabbit cornea. *Journal of Physiology*, **263**, 563–577

HOLDEN, B.A., BRENNAN, N.A., EFRON, N. *et al.* (1987) The contact lens: physiological considerations. In *Contact Lenses* (ed. J.V. Aquavella and G.N. Rao) Lippincott, Philadelphia, p. 4

HOLDEN, B.A. and SWARBRICK, H.A. (1987) Contact lens induced corneal oedema. In *The CLAO Guide to Basic Science and Clinical Practice* (ed. O. Dabezies Jr), 1984, Vol 1 Update II, Grune and Stratton, New York and London, pp. 15.6–15.15

HOLDEN, B., SWEENEY, D.F. and SANDERSON, G. (1984) The minimum precorneal oxygen tension to avoid corneal oedema. *Investigative Ophthalmology and Visual Science*, **25**, 476–480

HOLLY, F.J. (1987) Tear film physiology. *International Ophthalmology Clinics*, **27**, 2–6

JONES, D., LIVESY, S. and WILKINS, P. (1987) Hard contact lens migration into the upper lid: an unexpected lid lump. *British Journal of Ophthalmology*, **71**, 368–370

JORDAN, A. and BAUM, J.L. (1980) Basic tear flow–Does it exist? *Ophthalmology*, **87**, 920–930

KLYCE, S.D., FARRIS LINSY, and R. DABEZIES, O. JR. (1984) Corneal oxygenation in contact lens wearers. *CLAO Guide to Basic Science and Clinical Practice* (ed. O. Dabezies Jr), Vol 1, Grune and Stratton, New York and London, pp. 14.1–5

LANG, M.A. and HAMILL, J.R. (1973) Factors affecting the break-up time in normal eyes. *Archives of Ophthalmology*, **89**, 103–105

MCMONNIES, C. (1984) Contact lens induced corneal vascularisation. *The Journal of the British Contact Lens Association*, **7**, 154–157

MANDELL, R.B. and FARRELL, R. (1980) Corneal swelling at low atmospheric oxygen pressures. *Investigative Ophthalmology and Visual Science*, **19**, 697–702

MAURICE, D. (1972) Location of the fluid pump in the cornea. *Journal of Physiology*, **221**, 43–54

O'NEAL, M., POLSE, K. and SARVER, M. (1984) Corneal response to rigid and hydrogel lenses during eye closure. *Investigative Ophthalmology and Visual Science*, **25**, 837–842

POLSE, K. and MANDELL, R. (1970) Critical oxygen tension at the corneal surface. *Archives Opthalmology*, **84**, 505–508

SMELSER, G. and CHEN, D. (1955) Physiological changes in the cornea induced by contact lenses. *Archives Ophthalmology*, **53**, 676–679

THOFT, R. and FRIEND, J. (1975) Biochemical aspects of contact lens wear. *American Journal of Ophthalmology*, **80**, 139–145

WILSON, M.S. (1971) Corneal oedema from corneal contact lens wear, its cause and treatment. *Transactions of the Ophthalmic Society of the United Kingdom*, **XL**, 31–45

Bacteriology

CREMONS, C.S., COHEN, E.J., ARENTSEN, J.J., *et al.* (1987) *Pseudomonas* ulcers following patching of corneal abrasions. *The CLAO Journal*, **13**, 161–164

COHEN, E.J., PARLATO, C.J., ARENTSEN, J.J., *et al.* (1987) Medical and surgical treatment of Acanthamoeba keratitis. *American Journal of Ophthalmology*, **103**, 615–626

DEPARTMENT of HEALTH and SOCIAL SECURITY (1986) *LAV/HTLV III the Causative Agent of AIDS and Related Conditions. Revised Guidelines*, HMSO, London

DIXON, J. (1964) Ocular changes due to contact lenses. *American Journal of Optometry*, **58**, 424–443

DURAN, J.A., REFOJO, M.F., GIPSON, I.K., *et al.* (1987) Pseudomonas attachment to new hydrogel contact lenses. *Archives of Ophthalmology*, **105**, 106–109

EASTY, D.L. (1988) Acanthamoeba keratitis. *British Medical Journal*, **296**, 228

FACULTY OF OPHTHALMOLOGISTS (1986) Advice to British Ophthalmologists on AIDS. *Journal British Contact Lens Association; Scientific meetings report* 28

GALENTINE, P., COHEN, E., LAIBSON, P., *et al.* (1984) Corneal ulcers associated with contact lens wear. *Archives Ophthalmology*, **102**, 891–894

HASSMAN, G. and SUGAR, J. (1983) *Pseudomonas* corneal ulcer with extended wear soft contact lenses for myopia. *Archives Ophthalmology*, **101**, 1549–1550

KAPETANSKY, F., SUIE, T. and GRACY, D., *et al.* (1964) Bacteriologic studies of patients who wear contact lenses. *American Journal of Ophthalmology*, **57**, 255–258

KOENIG, S.B., SOLOMON, J.M., HYNDIUK, R.A., *et al.* (1987) Acanthamoeba Keratitis associated with gas-permeable contact lens wear. *American Journal of Ophthalmology*, **103**, 832

MCCLELLAN, K. and COSTER, D.J., (1987) Acanthamoebic keratitis diagnosed by paracentesis and biopsy and treated with propamidine. *British Journal of Ophthalmology*, **71**, 734–736

MANNIS, M., TAMARIN, R., ROTH, A., *et al.* (1986) Acanthamoeba sclerokeratitis. *Achives Ophthalmology*, **104**, 1313–1317

ORMEROD, D. and SMITH, R. (1986) Contact lens-associated microbial keratitis. *Archives Ophthalmology*, **104**, 79–83

SLUSHER, M., MYRNVIK, Q., LEWIS, J., *et al.* (1987) Extended-wear lenses, biofilm and bacterial adhesion. *Archives of Ophthalmology*, **105**, 110–115

TERVO, T., LANDEVIRTA, J., VEHERI, A., *et al.* (1986) Recovery of HTLV III from contact lenses *The Lancet*, February 15, 379–380

U.S. FOOD and DRUG ADMINISTRATION (1986) Recommendations for preventing the possible transmission of Human-T-lymphocyte virus Type III/lymphadenopathy-associated virus from tears. *Journal British Contact Lens Association: Scientific meetings report* 28–29

VOGT, M., HO, D. and BAKAR, S., *et al*, (1986) Safe disinfection of contact lenses after contamination with HTLV III. *Ophthalmology*, **93**, 771–773

WILSON, L. and AHEARN, D. (1986) Association of fungi with extended wear contact lenses. *American Journal of Ophthalmology*, **101**, 434–

WINKLER, C. and DIXON, J. (1964) Bacteriology of the eye III A. Effect of contact lenses on the normal flora B. Flora of the contact lens case. *Archives Ophthalmology*, **72**, 817–819

3

Contact lens manufacture, materials and types

The search for contact lenses with fewer problems and more comfort has resulted in the development of many new materials. This chapter will describe the various lens types, the important properties of the materials used to make contact lenses and broad guidelines on the interpretation of manufacturers data sheets.

Contact lenses are made from polymers, consisting of a large number of repeating subunits of monomer, or co-polymers, which contain two or more chemically different monomers. In order to stabilize the co-polymer, cross-linkages are usually incorporated into the molecule.

Methods of manufacture

Rigid lenses

These may be lathe cut or moulded.

Lathe-cut lenses

This method allows all the parameters of a lens to be specified so that an individually designed lens is possible. Even after manufacture some adjustments are possible. A lathe-cut lens is usually made with a spherical back surface but it is now possible to make aspheric back curves.

Moulded lenses

Rigid corneal lenses can be made by moulding the polymer between quartz glass moulds, as in Wohlk's Parabolar and Hartflex lenses and sheets of polymer may be impression moulded to make scleral lenses.

Soft lenses

Lathe-cut lenses

Soft lenses are lathed in the dehydrated state and then hydrated under controlled conditions.

The disadvantage of this method of manufacture, for either type of lens, is that lenses are less reproducible. However the increasing use of automation, computer controlled lathes and better control of temperature and humidity in the laboratory increases reliability.

Moulded lenses

Cast or injection moulded lenses have good optical surfaces and are very reproducible, but are only made in limited parameters which cannot be altered. Vistakon disposable lenses are moulded from liquid monomer and are accurately reproducible.

Spuncast lenses

Soft lenses can be spuncast from liquid monomer. The lens is reliably reproducible with an optically good aspheric back surface and thin edges. The lenses tend to be comfortable with good wearing time. The power of the lens, unlike lathe-cut and moulded lenses, is determined by the back surface, and depends on the volume of monomer and the spin speed.

15

A combination of methods can be used, as in the Bausch and Lomb Optima 38 lens, which has a spuncast anterior surface and a lathe-cut posterior surface. The manufacturers claim that this results in a more rigid lens, which is easier to handle.

Properties of contact lens materials

A contact lens must be comfortable and should not cause damage to the eye. The material needs to be strong enough to withstand daily handling and must be stable, so that it retains its shape. Its refractive index should provide good vision and it should be simple to clean and sterilize. Four further features of contact lens materials are important and are considered in greater detail.

Wettability

For comfort and clear vision the surface of a contact lens needs to be wet. Fluids adhere to solids, forming a wetting angle (θ) (Figure 3.1).

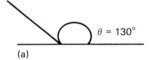
(a)

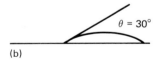
(b)

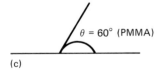
(c)

Figure 3.1   Diagram to show (a) large wetting angle with little spread of fluid over the solid surface, (b) low wetting angle with considerable wetting of the solid and (c) wetting angle of PMMA

On hydrophobic surfaces the forces between the fluid molecules attract one another and the water forms a drop (Figure 3.1a) but on hydrophilic surfaces the liquid spreads over the material (Figure 3.1b). Substances with small wetting angles are hydrophilic and those with large wetting angles are hydrophobic. Hydrophilic materials, with small wetting angles make the most comfortable contact lenses. The wetting angle of hydrophobic PMMA is 60°.

Gas transmission

Gas transmission is an important feature of modern contact lens materials, and refers to the ability of oxygen and carbon dioxide to pass through the lens. Three terms are in common use.

Oxygen permeability (Dk)

This is an intrinsic property of the material and is defined as

$$P = Dk \ (\text{cm}^2 \ \text{ml} \ O_2)/(\text{sec} \times \text{ml} \times \text{mmHg})$$

where P is the oxygen permeability coefficient of a material
D is the diffusion coefficient, and
k is the solubility coefficient.

Dk is dependent on temperature and is often quoted at room temperature instead of the more logical corneal temperature (35°C). However some degree of assessment can be made, using the former, as the higher the temperature, the higher the Dk value.

Dk is not dependent on the thickness of the material and therefore different materials can be compared, but it is less applicable to finished lenses. In PMMA and RGP materials the Dk value is a property of the plastic itself, but in soft lenses it is directly related to the water content of the material.

Materials with Dk values ranging from 2–92×10^{-11} are in clinical use with higher values being used experimentally.

Oxygen transmissibility (Dk/t)

This is the amount of oxygen that will diffuse through a lens in unit time, for a given oxygen tension.

Transmissibility = Dk/t (cm sec) $\times$ (ml O_2/ml)
material $\times$ mmHg)
where Dk is the gas permeability
t is the lens thickness

A contact lens varies in thickness, being thicker centrally than peripherally in a plus lens, and vice versa in a minus lens. These characteristics become more important with increasing powers but clinically it is generally sufficient to use the central thickness of a lens in calculations. Lenses with low Dk/t values may not provide sufficient oxygen at the cornea (Mandell, 1982), but with the help of the tear pump an adequate supply can be maintained by a lens of given thickness. There is little or no tear pump action during sleep so lenses with high Dk/t values are required for extended wear. It has been suggested that values as high as 75×10^{-9} are necessary to prevent oedema if a lens is worn during sleep (Polse and O'Neal, 1986). For Dk/t values see Appendix 6.

Equivalent oxygen percentage

This relates the percentage of oxygen available at the cornea to the percentage of atmospheric oxygen, on a scale of 0–21%, where 21% is equivalent to no lens on the eye. A reduction in EOP has been found when protein deposits build up on a lens (Hill, 1980) and values also alter with lens thickness (Hill, 1982).

Hydration

All lenses will absorb some water. This is minimal with PMMA, but is approximately 2% for RGP materials. However the soft lens materials can absorb between 25–79% by weight of water. Lenses with a high water content have a high Dk value and are less stable dimensionally. They are more difficult to handle but may be more comfortable to wear.

Soft lenses lose water by evaporation when on the eye. In a patient with a reduced or abnormal tear film, the lens can tighten and cause discomfort. If soft lenses are left out of storage solution they will rapidly dehydrate and shrink. They can be rehydrated successfully, in sterile N-saline solution, if handled carefully.

Hardness

Adequate hardness is necessary for manufacturing accuracy, stability of the material and scratch resistance. Manufacturers use a variety of methods to evaluate hardness which makes comparison of materials difficult. All lenses will show some evidence of insignificant, superficial scratches. Rigid, lathed lenses can be repolished but may need replacing if the scratches are deep. RGP lenses are more prone to scratching than PMMA lenses.

Types of contact lens

There are three main classes of contact lens (see Table 3.1). Their advantages and disadvantages are summarized in Tables 3.2, 3.3 and 3.4.

PMMA lenses

PMMA is a polymer of monomethylmethacrylate (MMA). It has been in use since the 1940s and is also known, in the UK, as Perspex. PMMA is stable and biologically inert but has a hydrophobic surface with a high wetting angle, unless the surface is treated with a wetting agent. It has a minimal water content and is impermeable to oxygen. PMMA lenses are not suitable for intermittent wear because if they are not worn regularly tolerance is lost and must be rebuilt. They provide good vision, are useful for patients with astigmatic corneas, and are less likely to develop deposits than other types of lenses. PMMA is used to make scleral and prosthetic lenses.

Rigid gas-permeable lenses (RGP)

These are the most recent development in contact lens technology. They are similar in appearance to PMMA lenses and cannot, clinically, be differentiated from them in most cases, but some materials are a distinctive colour. There are five types of RGP lens (Table 3.1).

Table 3.1 Classification of contact lenses

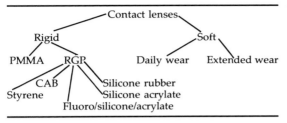

Table 3.2 Advantages and disadvantages of PMMA lenses

Advantages	Disadvantages
Gives good vision	Hydrophobic
Corrects astigmatism	Not gas permeable
Easy to maintain	Less comfortable
Long lasting	Not for intermittent
Less easily damaged	wear
Small thin lenses can be	Long adaptation period
made	Thin lenses break easily
Moulded scleral lenses	
possible	
Fit with fluoroscein	

Table 3.3 Advantages and disadvantages of RGP lenses

Advantages	Disadvantages
Good oxygen transmission	Lens flexure with high Dk/t
Greater comfort	Hydrophobic surfaces
Shorter adaptation time	More prone to deposits
Longer wearing time	Some are surface treated
Correct astigmatism	More fragile
Possibility of extended wear	
Fit with fluorescein	

Table 3.4 Advantages and disadvantages of soft lenses

Advantages	Disadvantages
Short adaptation period	Less good vision
More comfortable	Greater incidence infection
Good oxygen transmission	Deposits++
More stable on the eye	Shorter life span
Useful for intermittent wear	Easier to damage
Therapeutic uses	Absorbs toxic substances
Useful for babies	Do not correct astigmatism
	More expensive to buy
	More expensive to
	maintain
	Cannot use fluorescein

Cellulose acetate butyrate lenses (CAB)

CAB is a polymer that varies, depending on the number of acetyl or butyryl groups substituted for hydroxyl groups in the molecule. Therefore not all CAB materials behave in the same way. CAB has a low water content (2%) and a Dk value of 5×10^{-11} (Ratkowski, 1982). The problem with these lenses is the lack of cross-linking to stabilize the molecule so the lenses may warp. However this is not a significant problem under normal conditions. These lenses helped to reduce the problem of hypoxic corneal oedema. Since then manufacturers have sought to produce materials with increased oxygen permeability (see below).

Silicone/acrylate lenses

Silicone can be used as the siloxanyl radical with MMA, as in the Polycon lens (Pilkington Syntex Ophthalmics), as silicone radicals or as the rubbery elastomer siloxane. Silicone is highly oxygen permeable but very hydrophobic and any material incorporating it in the molecule will not wet well. To improve the wettability some manufacturers add hydrophilic substances such as methacrylic acid (MA) to the polymer. The silicone/acrylate lenses are an expanding group and include the Boston II and IV lenses (Polymer Technology) and the XL range of materials (Progressive Chemical Research).

Silicone rubber lenses

Unlike other RGP lenses as they are soft and elastic and the lens surface has to be specially treated to improve wettability. This makes it impossible to alter the lens or repolish the surface and to maintain the surface the lens must be stored in solution. The lens is permeable to water vapour, from the tears under the lens, which evaporate from the surface, resulting in a valve-like action when blinking, causing the lens to stick to the eye. These lenses are resistant to bacterial colonization and are useful as therapeutic lenses (Woodward, 1984). At the present time the only silicone lens available in the UK is the Wohlk Silflex lens. In the USA a similar lens is also made by Danker.

Styrene lenses

The Airlens (Wesley Jessen) is made from t-butyl styrene. It does not contain silicone but has a *Dk* value of 25×10^{-11} at 35°C. However there are some problems in caring for these lenses which are not suitable for heat sterilization or cleaning with Boston Cleaner, and chlorhexidine reduces its wettability.

Fluoropolymers

The newest group of RGP lenses are the fluoropolymers which have high *Dk* values. This group includes the Boston Equalens (Polymer Technology) with a *Dk* of 72×10^{-11} which is made from fluoro/siloxanyl/acrylate polymer and contains an ultraviolet light absorber, the Optacryl Z lens (Optacryl Inc.) with a *Dk* of 82×10^{-11} and the FluoroPerm lens (Paragon Optical International) with a *Dk* of 92×10^{-11}. These lenses are suitable for periods of extended wear (Gasson and Port, 1986) but the material flexes more readily on the eye (Rosenthal, 1986) and a temporary seal may form at the lens periphery when blinking (see Chapter 9). RGP lens materials are a compromise between increased oxygen transmission and wettability with a constant search being made for ways to increase the former without reducing the latter.

Soft lenses

Soft lenses have water contents which range between 25% and 79% and are subdivided into low water content lenses (below 50%) and high water content lenses (above 50%), with corresponding gas permeability. In the USA hydrophilic lens materials have the suffix -filcon, and hydrophobic lenses the suffix -focon.

There are two classes of soft lenses. Those made from polyhydroxyethylmethacrylate (pHEMA) and those which are non-HEMA lenses.

pHEMA lenses

pHEMA absorbs water and the parameters of a lens are only correct when the lens is fully hydrated in N-saline. The molecule is stabilized with cross-linkages, often of ethylene-glycol-dimethacrylate (EGDMA), and, to increase the water content may be co-polymerized with poly-vinylpyrrolidone (PVP) or *N*-vinylpyrrolidone.

Non-HEMA lenses

Some lenses are made without pHEMA, although the properties are similar, for example MMA and vinylpyrrolidone are used in Wohlk's Geaflex lens, and CLM's Sauflon lens consists of MMA and NVP cross-linked with EGDMA. The increasing variety of materials now available makes it possible to fit almost all patients satisfactorily.

References

GASSON, A. and PORT, M. (1986) Hard fluoropolymer lenses for extended wear. *Transactions of the British Contact Lens Association Annual Clinical Conference*, 39–43

HILL, R. (1980) The great oxygen race. *Contact Lens Journal*, **9**, 3–5

HILL, R. (1982) Oxygen: Passage through the periphery. *Contact Lens Journal*, **10**, 13–13

MANDELL, R. (1982) Corneal physiology and permeable materials. *Contact Lens Journal*, **10**, 9–15

POLSE, K.A. and O'NEAL, M.R. (1986) Oxygen requirements for extended wear. *The Journal of the British Contact Lens Association, Scientific meetings report*, 19–20

RATKOWSKI, D. (1982) Chemistry of cellulose acetate butyrate. *Contact Lens Journal*, **10**, 20

ROSENTHAL, P. (1986) Rigid superpermeable contact lenses. *Transactions of The British Contact Lens Association Annual Clinical Conference*, 88–90

WOODWARD, E.G. (1984) Therapeutic silicone rubber lenses. *Journal of the British Contact Lens Association*, **7**, 39–40

4

Contact lens care

All contact lenses are liable to accumulate secretions from the eye, substances transferred from the fingers when handling the lens, and cosmetics. RGP and soft lenses tend to develop deposits consisting of cell debris and protein, lipid and insoluble salts from the tear film. Lenses can also act as carriers of bacteria, viruses and fungi. To reduce the risk to the eye, and to prevent damage to the lens, the lens must be cleaned and stored correctly.

Solutions are available which care for the different types of lenses. Rigid lens solutions are unsuitable for soft lenses because their preservatives may bind to the lenses or cause a toxic reaction (see below). Some RGP solutions are unsuitable for lenses with specially treated surfaces, because they contain granular cleaning agents which can damage them. Solutions are usually marketed as 'sets' of cleaning, disinfecting and wetting/comfort solutions but some, such as Total (Allergan) and Contactasol Complete Care (Ciba Vision Contactasol), are multifunctional and can be used for all purposes. These solutions are simple to use, less expensive and easier to carry when travelling. However they may not be so effective as each solution used individually (Stein and Slatt, 1984) but many patients have used them satisfactorily for considerable periods.

Properties of solutions

Solutions which come into contact with the eye must be sterile and chemically stable from the time of manufacture throughout the period of storage

and use. They should not irritate or damage the eye or lens and, for comfort, they should be isotonic. Since January 1980 contact lens solutions in the UK have been controlled under the Medicines Act and are now marked with an expiry date and their contents.

Preservatives

To maintain their sterility, contact lens solutions contain preservatives, and these antimicrobials are the effective agents in most contact lens disinfecting solutions. They should be active against a wide range of organisms, including fungi and should not cause allergic or toxic reactions. The commonly used preservatives are:

1. Benzalkonium chloride (BKC)
2. Chlorbutanol (CHB)
3. Thiomersal (thimerosal) (THM)
4. Chlorhexidine (CHX)
5. Chelating agents
6. Sorbic acid or potassium sorbate

These preservatives are commonly used in eye drops and experience has shown that they should not harm the eye. However, as contact lens solutions are often in contact with the eye over long periods, particularly with soft lenses which absorb them, weaker concentrations are used (see Appendix 7).

Benzalkonium chloride (BKC)

The commonest preservative in hard lens solutions is BKC. It is effective over a wide range of

20

organisms (Hale, 1978) but is less effective against *Serratia marcesens* than *Pseudomonas* (Wilson, 1984). BKC is bacteriostatic and its effectiveness is reduced by soap, sponge and rubber which should be excluded from contact lens cases. It is unsuitable for use with soft lenses as it binds to the lens and has a toxic action on the corneal epithelium. BKC may also bind to RGP lenses (Rosenthal *et al.*, 1986) and the possibility should be considered in any patient with irritable eyes.

Chlorbutanol (CHB)

It is bactericidal and fungicidal but is slow acting. It is present in Liquifilm Tears (Allergan) and Blink n Clean (Allergan).

Chlorhexidine digluconate (CHX)

This highly effective preservative is used with rigid lenses but is rapidly absorbed and concentrated by soft lenses (Meakin, 1984) and toxic reactions may occur when the concentrated solution is released into the tears.

Thiomersal (thimerosal in USA) (THM)

Thiomersal is an effective antifungal and bactericidal agent (McTaggart, 1980) but it has a slow kill rate and can cause sensitivity reactions. These occur most often with soft lenses, but can occur with all types of lens. Thiomersal has been shown to cause a hypersensitivity reaction affecting the upper cornea and adjacent limbal area. There is a non-specific conjunctivitis with limbal follicles, corneal infiltrates and a punctate epithelial keratopathy together with superficial neovascularization (Wilson, 1980; Wilson, McNatt and Reitschel, 1981).

Chelating agents

Ethylene diamine tetracetic acid (EDTA) and disodium edetate have no active preservative action of their own but enhance the action of other compounds.

Sorbic acid

Sorbic acid and potassium sorbate preserved solutions are available for soft lens care but there have been reports of soft lens discolouration. This appears to be due to amines in the tear fluid reacting with degradation products of sorbic acid and discolouring lens deposits but the lens itself is clear (Sibley and Chu, 1984). The problem may be prevented by thorough cleaning of the lens, by not mixing solutions, nor heating the lens excessively. If discolouration does occur the lens should be cleaned professionally.

PMMA corneal lens care

The object of rigid lens care is to clean and disinfect the lens and to prevent damage to the lens or the eye. PMMA lenses are hydrophobic and are less affected by deposit formation than other types of lens.

Cleaning

Lenses should be cleaned daily, immediately on removal from the eye. This prevents contaminants such as grease, cosmetics and mucus drying and adhering to the lens surface. There are several methods of cleaning a lens.

Mechanical friction and a surfactant cleaner

A drop of cleaning solution is placed on the lens and the surface contaminants removed by rubbing the lens gently between the thumb and forefinger, taking care not to distort the lens. Surfactants will remove grease and cosmetics as well as protein film and salts. Miraflow (Ciba Vision Contactasol) is an effective, self-preserving cleaner, containing 20% isopropyl alcohol, without the usual preservatives.

The tip of a good quality artists brush (No 7), first wetted then shaken dry, can be used by the patient, with one drop of cleaning solution to clean both lens surfaces. This produces plenty of foam which is highly effective in cleaning the lens. It is very useful with lenticular lenses as dirt, mucus and dried solution can accumulate at the junction of the lenticular portion and the peripheral carrier. It is always difficult to clean this area well with fingers and is more difficult for the elderly aphakic with poor vision and loss of digital sensation. For the clinician it is preferable to use disposable cotton-wool buds, using a separate bud

for each lens, to prevent cross-infection, but it is not so effective.

Hydrodynamic cleaning (Figure 4.1)

With the Hydramat II (Barnes Hind) the lenses are placed in baskets, in a case containing cleaning solution. The case has a cap which rotates the baskets in the solution. This is done for 30 seconds and the movement of the solution loosens any deposits.

The SOFTMATE Professional Cleaning Unit (Barnes-Hind) is a device which produces high energy vibrations which are transmitted into the Hydra-Mat II case. It produces a standing wave of cleaning solution in the case which cleans the lens.

Ultrasonic cleaning

This is used by manufacturers and in the practice and is very efficient but is generally too expensive for home use, although smaller, cheaper units are becoming available.

Cleaning solutions are not designed to be used in the eye. They are stronger than disinfecting or wetting solutions and should be rinsed off the lens after use. The patient may, however, inadvertently use them in the eye and, whilst these solutions may cause a transient keratitis, they do not usually result in lasting damage.

Lens greasing may be improved by using a cleaner such as Miraflow which is effective against lipids.

Disinfection

Cleaned lenses are not sterile and need to be disinfected. The lenses are placed in a soaking/disinfecting solution overnight or for a minimum of five hours. An ideal soaking solution should have a wide spectrum of activity, including *Pseudomonas*, and should be fungicidal.

Buffering these solutions stabilizes the pH and helps to maintain their effectivity (Davies, 1980).

Lens storage

Lenses are stored in plastic containers which are designed to minimize damage. The baskets holding the lens must be deep enough to allow the lens to be completely covered with disinfecting/soaking solution. Mailing cases are not adequate as the volume of solution contained is insufficient to prevent the lens from drying out. The design of the case and baskets should make regular cleaning easy (Figure 4.2).

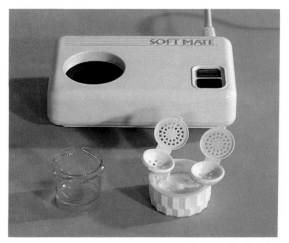

Figure 4.1 Hydrodynamic cleaning; Barnes Hind soft lens case and Softmate soft lens cleaner

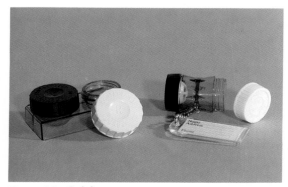

Figure 4.2 Soft lens cases

Lenses are stored in solution as the lens is cleaner, more comfortable when placed on the eye and gives better vision. The solution also provides a cushion which prevents lens damage.

Patients should understand that cases, as well as lenses, need regular cleaning, as they are often the source of infection.

Wetting solutions

PMMA lenses are hydrophobic and the wetting angle can be reduced by a wetting solution which produces an even spread of tear film over the lens and increased comfort. Wetting solutions contain a preservative, wetting and buffering agents, methylcellulose and sodium chloride. The common wetting agents are polyvinylpyrrolidone (PVP) and polyvinyl alcohol (PVA). Wetting solutions are useful as an aid to inserting the lens, as their greater viscosity helps the lens to adhere to the finger when placing the lens on the eye.

Detailed instructions for the care of lenses are to be found in Chapters 7 and 8.

Rigid gas-permeable lens care

The same routine of cleaning, disinfecting and wetting is used for RGP lenses as for PMMA lenses. However the 2% water content of these lenses and their more delicate surfaces mean that if they are allowed to dry their parameters will alter and, as the plastic is softer than PMMA, they easily become scratched. They should always be stored in solution to keep the lens hydrated.

RGP lens cleaning and disinfection

RGP lenses are more affected by deposit formation than PMMA lenses, but less affected than soft lenses. Deposits are due to the negative ionic charge on the lens surface attracting positively charged ions from the tear film. They form as a milky/brown film of protein, or as wart like deposits which consist of lipid, particularly cholesterol, and salts, often occurring as a peripheral ring on the surface of the lens. Solutions specifically designed for use with RGP lenses are now available. The cleaning solution of the Boston Care System (Polymer Technology), coats the lens so that it is more hydrophilic and alters the surface charge making the lens less attractive to deposits. The solution also contains a 'friction enhancing agent' to help remove deposits. A similar solution, Concentrated Cleaner (Bausch and Lomb), contains 'polymeric beads'.

Protein removing tablets (see below) can be used routinely each week, to clean the lens, but it is preferable to assess the new wearer and adopt a regime appropriate to the individual, depending on the time taken to build up deposits. Some patients need to use them every one or two weeks, others monthly and some never. This variation appears to be related to any tendency to dry eyes, the effectivity of blinking and the care with which the lens is cleaned daily. The lens should be stored in RGP disinfecting/soaking solution.

Soft contact lens care

The two main problems experienced with soft lenses are their tendency to form deposits and to discolour.

Deposits

These form as an even coat of surface film, due to protein, or as discrete, circular, sometimes berry-like elevations and are a major problem. They consist of muco-proteins and lipids, particularly cholesterol, together with calcium salts and cell debris. They occur more often in dry eyes, with altered tear film, with damaged lenses and particularly if there have been previous deposits on the lens.

Deposits cause reduced vision as the lens gradually becomes opaque, with reduced oxygen transmissability leading to hypoxia and discomfort. They may also cause irritation due to absorbed chemicals. Large deposits cause mechanical irritation as the lids pass over them and there is increased lens movement as the upper lids adhere to them, causing the lens to move with the blink, resulting in variable vision. The Hydrocurve Elite lens (Barnes Hind) has been designed with a surface which is, ionically, almost neutral. This

reduces the attraction of deposits for the lens and facilitates their removal.

Deposits should not be allowed to build up on the lens, as the larger the deposit the more difficult it is to remove. An affected lens may be sent to a laboratory for cleaning. As a charge is made for this the lens should be carefully examined for any damage, as it will then need replacing. Cleaned lenses should be examined to ensure that all the deposit has been successfully removed. If some residual deposit remains the lens may be used, providing it does not cause symptoms, until a new lens is obtained.

Discolouration

Discolouration usually occurs with soft lenses.

Local causes

1. Topical sources of discolouration include neutral adrenaline (epinephrine USA) eye-drops which turn the lenses brown/black. Drops and contact lens solutions which are preserved with sorbic acid or potassium sorbate may turn the lenses yellow, particularly with heat disinfection. Chlorhexidine may make them yellow/green and soft lenses tend to yellow with age.
2. Fungal hyphae may penetrate the lens matrix and produce surface growths which may be heavily pigmented.

Systemic causes

Orange discolouration has been reported with rifampicin (Harris and Jenkins, 1985) and yellow lenses occurred from sulphasalazine (Riley, Flegg and Mandel, 1986)

Miscellaneous causes

These include tobacco smoke which can turn the lens yellow and make-up which can result in a variety of colours.

Soft lens cleaning

Cleaning is more complex and more expensive for soft lenses than for other types of lens.

Surfactants

These lower surface tension and so remove traces of grease, cosmetics and a certain amount of protein. The lenses are cleaned by rubbing both surfaces gently with a finger and thumb, to loosen contaminants. Alternatively the lens may be cleaned using a finger with the lens in the palm of the hand, for the inner surface and on the middle finger, for the front surface. Care must be taken not to damage the lens. Some cleaning solutions, such as Sauflon Soft Lens Daily Cleaner (Sauflon Pharmaceuticals Limited) contain hypertonic saline which shrinks the lens and loosens surface adherents (Healey, 1982). Pliagel (Alcon) is a soft lens cleaner preserved with sorbic acid as is Sensitive Eyes Daily Cleaner (Bausch and Lomb).

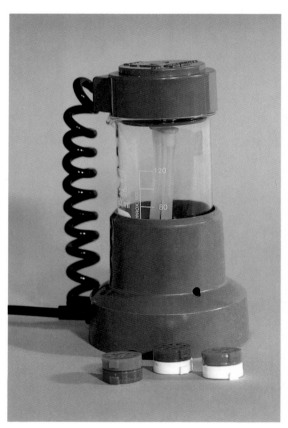

Figure 4.3 Magnetic stirrer (Focus). Soft contact lenses are placed, in the baskets, in solution containing an oxidising agent and heated at a constant temperature for 2 hours.

Enzyme systems

Enzyme systems are used to remove protein deposits from soft and RGP lenses. Hydrocare Fizzy (Allergan) contains the enzyme papain which dissolves the protein deposit, but care must be taken to rinse the lens well, as any residual enzyme may cause an irritated, red eye.

Amiclair (Abatron) contains two proteases and a lipase but, no papain, and is claimed to remove protein, lipid and mucus.

Softmate Protein Remover solution (Barnes Hind) is available in the USA and is supplied as unit dose containing boric acid.

Following enzyme treatment the lenses must be rinsed and disinfected in the normal way.

Oxidation systems

The principle of these systems is that oxidation of the deposits results in water soluble substances which can then be removed by rinsing.

Liprofin (Burton Parsons) and Monoclens (Sauflon Pharmaceuticals) contain sodium perborate which produces oxygen on heating (Phillips, 1980). The lenses are heated in the solution for two hours, in a magnetic stirrer (Figure 4.3) which maintains a temperature of 60–70°C, after which they are rinsed then autoclaved in N-saline in sealed containers.

Disinfection

Soft lenses may be disinfected by heat or by chemicals.

Heat disinfection

Lenses disinfected by heat are pasteurized, as the temperatures obtained are not adequate for true sterilization. Always check to make sure that the lens is suitable for heat disinfection.

The lenses should be cleaned thoroughly, prior to disinfection, to remove the protein film. If cleaning is inadequate any protein remaining on the lens will be denatured by the heat and cannot be removed. Denatured protein may cause an allergic conjunctivitis.

Electric heating units are available which heat the lens, in saline, to the required temperature for a given period and then switch off automatically.

The units are more expensive than other methods but are more reliable. Lenses may be heated by boiling in buffered, unpreserved N-saline, and vacuum flasks filled with boiling water have also been used (Kuttner, Hamilton and Pennington, 1974). The lenses are heated in cases designed to withstand the temperature. Commercially prepared sterile saline is preferred as saline prepared from salt tablets and distilled water has been found to be the source of infection (Wilson, 1984).

Heat as a means of sterilization is adequate, the running costs are low and it avoids chemical reactions but the lifespan of the lens is reduced. Where there is a risk of *Acanthamoeba* infection, it is preferable that low water content lenses (less than 45% water) are heat sterilized; high water content lenses may be chemically disinfected, but there may be a greater risk of infection. If high water content lenses are heated they may need to be replaced more often (CLAO Policy Statement, 1988).

Chemical disinfection

Chemical disinfection is effective and easily portable. Until recently the most commonly used disinfecting agents were those used for rigid lens solutions, with the exception of benzalkonium chloride, which binds to soft lenses, and chlorhexidine which concentrates in soft lenses. An attempt has been made with Pryme solutions (Smith and Nephew) to minimize this effect by manufacturing solutions with lower concentrations of chlorhexidine. The most common solution reaction is to thiomersal (see above) and solutions containing this preservative are best avoided, particularly in any patient with a history of allergy or solution sensitivity.

To minimize sensitivity reactions, manufacturers have concentrated on designing regimes without preservatives. There are two substances in use at the present time.

Chlorine

In the Softabs system (Alcon) chlorine is released when a tablet of sodium dichloroisocyanurate is dissolved in 10 ml of unpreserved N-saline. The lens is soaked overnight, or for a minimum of four hours.

In the Aerotab system (Sauflon Pharmaceuticals) chlorine is released by a halozone tablet in N-saline. The lens should be soaked for at least 30 minutes or overnight.

After disinfecting with either system the lens should be rinsed with unpreserved N-saline before inserting it in the eye. The advantages of these systems are that they do not contain preservatives, the procedure can be carried out in a single container, there is no neutralization and they are suitable for use with trial lens sets (see Chapter 2). Elderly patients find the single stage procedure less confusing than the more complicated regimes.

Hydrogen peroxide

Hydrogen peroxide 3% will clean and disinfect soft lenses. The peroxide remaining in the lens and solution after the procedure is complete must then be neutralized. This can be done by photo-reduction, catalysis, chemicals or biological methods. Failure to neutralize residual peroxide results in discomfort but no lasting damage to the eye.

In the Septicon system (Ciba Vision Contactasol) the lens is disinfected for 20 minutes in Lensept, a 3% hydrogen peroxide solution (Janoff, 1979). The lens is then transferred to a separate container containing Lensrins (N-saline) and a platinum disc to neutralize the residual peroxide. Although the Lensept is unpreserved, the Lensrins is marketed, in the UK, with thiomersal as the preservative. In cases of thiomersal sensitivity this may be replaced by unpreserved saline. In other countries Lensrins is available without thiomersal as the preservative.

With the Contactasol 10:10 system (Ciba Vision Contactasol) the lens is soaked in 3% hydrogen peroxide for 10 minutes followed by 10 minutes neutralization in sodium pyruvate and N-saline solution (Billig *et al.*, 1984). It is preferable to extend the soaking time in each solution to 15 minutes, but no longer in the hydrogen peroxide as it makes the lens swell. It is also preferable to leave the lens overnight in the neutralizing solution so that the lens can return to its normal parameters or it may be uncomfortable to wear. This system is quicker with only a single container, which is also cleaned and disinfected by the hydrogen peroxide.

Oxysept (Allergan) is another 3% hydrogen peroxide system, the neutralizer is the enzyme catalase. These solutions are free from preservative but the starter packs are marketed with LC65 as the lens cleaner which contains thiomersal.

Chemical disinfection costs less than heat initially but the annual running cost at the time of writing (1988) are approximately £150 for soft lenses. Nevertheless it is a more reliable method, lens life is longer and protein is less likely to be denatured. However chemicals may bind to the lenses causing irritation and sensitivity reactions.

Saline and contact lenses

Because of the contamination experienced when using salt tablets and distilled water to make saline, other alternatives were sought. Sterile N-saline can be purchased either preserved or unpreserved, buffered or unbuffered.

Unpreserved saline

This can be obtained as unit dose sachets, which ensure that the solution is not used repeatedly, but can be messy, or as multidose aerosols which are easy to use but are more expensive. Unpreserved saline is used for sterilization by heat and chemicals, for rinsing, and as a wetting solution in cases of allergy. Most new soft lenses are transported in sterile, unpreserved saline, packed in sealed vials.

Preserved saline

Preserved saline is available in plastic bottles, with and without a calcium deposit preventer incorporated in the solution. It may be used for heat sterilization.

Table 4.1 Lubricants for use in dry eyes

A. Containing hypromellose
   Isoptoalkaline (Alcon)
   Isoptoplain (Alcon)
   Tears Naturale with dextran (Alcon)
B. Containing polyvinylalcohol
   Hypotears (Ciba Vision Contactasol)
   Liquifilm Tears (Allergan)
   SnoTears (Smith & Nephew)

Saline rewetting eye drops

Unpreserved saline eye drops are useful for patients with sensitivity reactions and in soft lens wearers with dry eyes. They are available as a unit dose dropper e.g. Clerz (Ciba Vision Contactasol), or as 15 ml bottles of Softmate rewetting drops (Barnes Hind) which are preserved with potassium sorbate. Unpreserved saline is not available as eye drops, because of the risk of infection, except in very small quantities as Minims Saline.

Lubricating eye drops

Rigid lenses may become uncomfortable because there is insufficient tear film or increased mucus secretion. Lubricating drops containing hypromellose, polyvinyl alcohol (Table 4.1) may be used and acetylcysteine 5% and hypromellose 0.35% (Ilube, Duncan Flockhart) are particularly useful for dry eyes with excessive mucus.

Choice of care system

The method selected to care for a lens depends on the type of lens, the tendency to form deposits and whether there is any history of sensitivity to solutions. An important factor is the ability of the patient to understand the steps necessary to care for the lens. A simple system is best for the young and the elderly who find that using a variety of solutions, and transferring lenses between containers, is confusing.

References

BILLIG, H., BAILEY, N., FLEISCHMAN, W., *et al*, (1984) A new, rapid hydrogen peroxide system for contact lens disinfection. *The CLAO Journal*, **10**, 341–345

CLAO POLICY STATEMENT (1988) Contact Lens Care; New Guidlines. *The CLAO Journal*, **14**, 55–56

DAVIES, D.J.G. (1980) Manufacture and supply of contact lens products *The Pharmaceutical Journal*, September 27, 343–345

HALE, R.H. (1978) Contact lens solutions. In *Contact Lenses. A clinical approach to fitting*, 1st edn, Williams and Wilkins, Baltimore, pp. 32–36

HARRIS, J. and JENKINS, P. (1985) Discolouration of soft contact lenses by rifampicin. *The Lancet*, November 16, 1133

HEALEY, J.N.C. (1982) A guide to contact lens care. *The Pharmaceutical Journal*, December 4, 650–654

JANOFF, L. (1979) Effective disinfection of soft contact lenses using hydrogen peroxide. *Contacto*, **23**, 37–40

KUTTNER, N.S., HAMILTON, W. and PENNINGTON, R.N. (1974) Sterilization of soft contact lenses using boiling water in a vacuum flask. *British Medical Journal*, **4**, 759–760

MCTAGGART, C. (1980) Care of soft contact lenses. *The Pharmaceutical Journal*, March 15, 309–313

MEAKIN, B. (1984) Contact lens solutions in the UK. *Journal of the British Contact Lens Association*, **7**, 192–203

PHILLIPS, A.J. (1980) The cleaning of hydrogel contact lenses. *Ophthalmic Optician*, May 24

RILEY, S.A., FLEGG, P.T. and MANDAL, B.K. (1986) Contact lens staining due to sulphasalazine. *The Lancet*, April 26, 972

ROSENTHAL, P., CHU, M.H., SALAMONE, J.C. and ISRAEL, S.C. (1986) Preservative interaction with GP lenses. *Optician*, **192**, No 5075, 33–38

SIBLEY, M.J. and CHU, V. (1984) Understanding sorbic acid-preserved contact lens solutions. *International Contact Lens Clinic*, **11**, 531–539

STEIN, H.A. and SLATT, B.J. (1984) *Fitting guide for rigid and soft contact lenses*, 2nd edn, The CV Mosby Company, St. Louis, Toronto, pp. 163–173

WILSON, L. (1980) Thiomersal hypersensitivity in soft contact lens wearers. *Contact Lens Journal*, **9**, 21–24

WILSON, L. (1984) Contact lens solutions in the US. *Journal British Contact Lens Association*, **7**, 213–217

WILSON, L., MCNATT, J. and REITSCHEL, R. (1981) Delayed hypersensitivity to thiomersal in soft contact lens wearers. *Ophthalmology*, **88**, 804–809

5

Equipping a contact lens practice

Contact lens fitting can be grouped into three main functions:

1. Assessment and fitting
2. Teaching
3. Lens inspection and verification

Assessment and fitting

Essential items are a slit-lamp, a keratometer and sets of trial contact lenses.

The slit-lamp

This is used at the initial visit to exclude any ocular contra-indications to contact lens wear and to assess the fit of the trial lens on the eye. During the follow-up period the effects of the lens on the eye are observed and the lens can be inspected.

The keratometer (ophthalmometer)

The keratometer measures the radius of curvature of the cornea, from which the refractive power of the cornea can be calculated, and scales in dioptres as well as millimetres radius of curvature are incorporated in the instruments. These readings provide a guide in selecting the initial trial lens and can be used to estimate the amount of corneal astigmatism. The keratometer can also be used to check the front and back radius of curvature of rigid contact lenses (see below). Several manual and automatic keratometers are available.

Manual keratometers

One or two-position instruments are available. They consist of a short-focus telescope, doubling devices and internally illuminated mires. The principle is based on the mires, acting as the extremities of an object of known angular size, being reflected by the cornea, which behaves as a convex mirror. The doubling device is usually one or two prisms and is used to make measurements easier and more accurate, despite the constant fine movements of the eye. The device results in three or four images, depending on the number of prisms. These images must be superimposed or aligned. To do this the mire separation can be altered while the power and position of the doubling device remain the same (fixed doubling), or the position of the device can be varied whilst the mire spearation remains the same (variable doubling). Fixed doubling occurs in instruments with single prisms and readings are taken in one meridian and then the instrument is moved through 90° to record the curvature of the other meridian. This is the two-position keratometer (Figure 5.1). Instruments with variable doubling have two prisms creating images in the horizontal and vertical meridia simultaneously and the instrument does not have to be moved to take the second reading (one-position instrument). Although this makes for rapid measurement, and corneal irregularities may be more obvious with the type of mire used, it can be difficult to align the instrument with the subjects eye.

Various designs of mires are used (Figure 5.2). Only the Javal Schiotz mires are coloured and this makes the end-point easier to see because overlapping of the colours produces white light.

There are potential sources of error which can be minimized when using a keratometer.

1. The images should be observed with both eyes open and with the observers accommodation relaxed.
2. The eyepiece should be correctly focused for the individual observer. This is done by rotating the eyepiece anticlockwise until the fine crosswire, visible through the eyepiece, is out of focus. The eyepiece is then rotated clockwise until the crosswire is clearly focused. The point on the eyepiece scale at which this happens is noted and, before using the instrument on subsequent occasions, the observer should check that the setting is correct. This is particularly important when instruments are shared.
3. The keratometer is designed to measure the radius of curvature of the cornea in millimetres and not as dioptric power. In the UK the former is the normal unit of measurement, but in some countries dioptric power is preferred. This may induce a small error as different models are calibrated using different indices to convert millimetres into dioptres. Either the Standard Index (1.3375) or the Tear Index (1.336) is used. Therefore a measurement in dioptres on one instrument may differ slightly from another.
4. An area of cornea 2.6–4.0 mm in diameter is measured, depending on the type of instrument used and the corneal curvature. A steep cornea will produce smaller images and a flat cornea larger ones. Paracentral areas can be measured by a keratometer termed a topogometer, which has a movable fixation light. This can be used to measure the size of the optic cap, by determining the point at which the central curvature begins to flatten, and the curvature of the upper corneal surface, in cases of keratoconus. The range of the keratometer can be increased, for flat or conical corneas, by placing an additional lens over the aperture (Stein and Slatt, 1984). When the cornea is irregular the reflection of the mires may be distorted and accurate measurement is difficult and sometimes impossible.
5. The accuracy of the instrument should be checked regularly by using a mounted metal or plastic spherical surface, of known radius of curvature.

Automated keratometers

The photokeratoscope was designed to increase the area of cornea measured and is based on the principle of the Placido disc. Rings of light are reflected from the cornea, photographed and

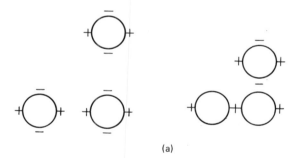

(a)

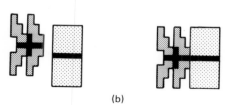

(b)

Figure 5.2 Keratometer mires (a) Bausch and Lomb type (b) Javal Schiotz mires as used in the Haag Streit keratometer

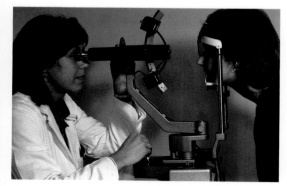

Figure 5.1 Haag Streit Keratometer

computer analysed. Accurate assessment is still difficult as the calculations depend on the measurement of the width between the rings, which are not always clearly defined. It is possible to adapt the Topcon photoslit-lamp for this purpose using the light source and built-in flash and a target of concentric rings, which are placed in front of the eye (Cotran and Miller, 1987).

The autokeratometer (Figure 5.3) is the latest development (Port, 1985). Readings can be taken over a larger area and the instrument will measure eccentric areas as well as the central curvatures. Rapid, accurate measurements are possible in most cases but it is difficult to obtain readings on highly astigmatic and irregular corneas, when it is still possible to record data from a manual instrument. The instrument also requires some patient co-operation and readings are not always possible in those with blepharospasm or head tremor.

Trial lenses

The most important factor in successful fitting is how the lens behaves on the eye. This is influenced by ocular factors as well as lens parameters. Trial lenses will show exactly how a given lens behaves on an individual patient, thus reducing the chances of an incorrectly fitting first lens, the number of visits needed and the subsequent cost of a replacement lens. In some practices inventory lenses are kept, which are large ranges of stock lenses, from which the patient can be both fitted and supplied. The advantage is that the patient

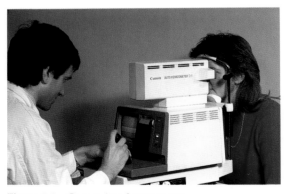

Figure 5.3   Canon Autokeratometer

can leave with their lenses after the initial visit. The disadvantage is that a large stock, requiring a large financial outlay, is necessary and some of the lenses in the range may never be used.

Uses of rigid trial lenses

To estimate the TD of the lens   An interpalpebral lens may cause discomfort and a lens which is too large may override the limbus when the patient looks down.

To assess the relationship of the back surface of the lens to the cornea using fluorescein. A lens which is too steep may be changed for a flatter lens and vice versa until the best fit is obtained (see Chapter 7).

To estimate visual acuity   An over refraction, with a contact lens on the eye, is more accurate with high refractive errors, when a spectacle refraction must allow for the back vertex distance. Very high myopes may achieve a better visual acuity with contact lenses than spectacles because there is less reduction in image size.

To obtain the best visual acuity with an irregular cornea   A rigid contact lens may be the only way of obtaining a good visual acuity. The liquid lens will neutralize the corneal irregularity, and the contact lens will correct any refractive error.

To estimate the best BOZR   When K-readings are impossible to obtain, in some cases of keratoconus and irregular corneae, trial lenses with different BOZRs can be used until a satisfactory fit is obtained.

Selection of fitting sets

Standard fitting sets are available from the manufacturers but it is preferable for the clinician to design his own. RGP lenses with low *Dk* values may be fitted using PMMA fitting sets, but the higher *Dk* value lenses need RGP fitting sets, because of their greater flexibility on the eye which decreases their ability to correct corneal astigmatism. PMMA and RGP sets are similar and are dealt with first under the same heading, although

PMMA lenses tend to be smaller and need more edge lift. Each lens parameter will now be considered.

Total diameter (TD) The total diameter, of a lens depends on the corneal diameter, width of the palpebral fissure and the fitting philosophy (see Chapter 7). The diameter of a rigid corneal lens must, by definition, be less than the cornea, and is uncomfortable should it cross the limbus during blinking or eye movements. RGP lenses can be a larger diameter than PMMA lenses as they are permeable to oxygen. Rigid lens diameters range from 7.0–12.0 mm, the most common being 8.5, 9.0, and 9.5 mm. Smaller lenses are less often used. For an initial trial set a TD of 9.0 mm is suggested. For aphakics 9.5 mm TD high plus lenses are better, as the larger TD stabilizes the heavy lens which centres better.

Back optic zone diameter (BOZD) This is the diameter of the 'fitting curve', the optic zone, of the lens. The BOZD is related to the TD, as sufficient width must be allowed for the peripheral curves, and to the size of the optic cap. BOZDs can range from 4.50 to 8.0 mm on a large lens when there is a large pupil or a broad iridectomy.

Back peripheral curves (BPC) The number of peripheral curves depends on the TD of the lens, the larger the lens the more peripheral curves are possible.

There are three methods of designing PCs for fitting sets. In the first the first back peripheral radius (FBPR) and the second back peripheral radius (SBPR), of a tri-curve lens, are flattened by a fixed amount, which is related to the BOZR. For example:

BOZR (BOZD)/ BOZR + 1.0 (FBPD)/ BOZR + 2.0 (TD)

so a lens with a radius of 7.8 would have the following specifications:

7.8 (7.5)/ 8.8 (8.5)/ 9.8 (9.5)

Some trial sets modify this so that there is a fixed increase on the FBPR but a constantly flat second radius as in

BOZR (BOZD)/ BOZR + 0.5 (FBPD)/ 2.0 (TD)

The second design of PCs uses constant axial edge lift (CAEL)(Stone and Francis, 1980). The axial edge lift (AEL) is the distance in millimetres, parallel to the lens axis, between the lens edge and the extrapolation of the BOZR (Figure 5.4). All lenses with CAEL will have similar peripheral clearances whereas, with a fixed relationship the edge lift varies with the steepness of the lens (Phillips, 1980).

The third method is that used by Atkinson and Kerr (1987) to design a trial set for the Boston Equalens. This uses constant axial edge clearance (CAEC). Axial edge clearance (AEC) (Figure 5.4) is the distance in millimetres, parallel to the lens axis, between the lens edge and the cornea. Atkinson showed that because some steep corneas flatten rapidly, and some flat corneas may similarly steepen, better edge clearance is obtained using the CAEC technique, and this is particularly applicable to highly gas-permeable lenses.

When trial sets are ordered the clinician may specify the type of edge clearance that is required. Suggested peripheral curves for PMMA trial sets are:

BOZR (7.5)/ BOZR + 1.3 (9.0) for a bi-curve lens
BOZR (7.5)/ BOZR + 0.5 (FBPD)/ BOZR + 1.0 (9.5) for a tri-curve lens.

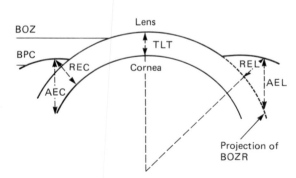

Figure 5.4 Peripheral curve design. The diagram shows the relationship between the peripheral curve of a lens and (a) the curve of the back optic zone, forming the edge lift and (b) the cornea–the edge clearance (BOZR, back optic zone radius; BOZ, back optic zone; BPC, back peripheral curve; TLT, tear layer thickness; REC, radial edge clearance; AEC, axial edge clearance; REL, radial edge lift, AEL, axial edge lift)

For RGP lenses:

BOZR (7.5)/ BOZR + 1.0 (9.0) for a bi-curve lens
BOZR (7.5)/ BOZR + 0.5 (FBPD)/ BOZR + 0.7 (9.5) for a tri-curve lens.

If a standard manufacturers trial set is used it is important to know which design method is used.

Back optic zone radius (BOZR)   A range of radii is needed for each fitting set. The most suitable for general use are a range from 7.2–8.5 mm in 0.1 mm steps. This must be discussed with the manufacturer when the sets are ordered, as otherwise 0.05 mm steps may be supplied. While these are sometimes useful it is possible to fit successfully with fewer lenses. Phillips (1980) used 0.05 mm steps for the middle of the range but 0.10 mm steps at either end. A set of lenses suitable for keratoconus is discussed in Chapter 12.

Soft lenses   These are larger than rigid corneal lenses and overlap the sclera. The commonest diameters are 13.0 and 13.5 mm, but may range from 12.50 to 15.50 mm. Daily wear soft lenses are available in different BOZRs, usually in 0.2 mm steps for pHEMA of average thickness, as the fit is less critical. Similarly thinner and high water content lenses are made in 0.3 mm and 0.4 mm steps, as two fits only (Steep and Flat) or even as One fit only. Each trial set contains a range of diameters and radii, as fewer lenses are needed.

All types of trial set need to have a range of powers available. Most low myopes and hypermetropes can be fitted using plano lenses and ±3.50 DS. High myopes and hypermetropes are better fitted using sets of ±7.0 DS and ±14.0 DS. The choice of these powers is significant, in order to keep any over refraction within 3.50 DS and so eliminate the problem of back vertex power.

Because of the large number of variables in lens fitting, a range of trial lenses makes fitting easier, but the beginner needs only the essential sets in a range of powers, which can be increased as needed. Eventually sets of special lenses including toric and bifocal lenses can be added.

Choice of manufacturer

Many contact lens manufacturers supply lenses to their own standard dimensions, and there is an extra charge for lenses outside these parameters.

Others make individual lenses to order, as well as making more complicated lenses.

The first consideration is the quality of lenses supplied. These should be consistently accurate with good edges, and the power and other parameters should be within their published tolerances. The manufacturer should offer a wide range of materials and parameters. Some companies have an exchange scheme for soft lenses.

Price is obviously a factor in purchasing lenses, but lenses may cost less because they are only supplied in a limited range, and are not exchangeable, so it is necessary to read the advertising material carefully. Finally the location of the manufacturer may have a bearing on the choice of supplier. Lenses made abroad may have to be imported, causing delay. Some firms will collect and deliver lenses daily in their own locality.

Ultraviolet lamp (Burton lamp)

This is a lamp consisting of fluorescent tubes of ultraviolet, and sometimes also white light, mounted in a holder with a +5.00 DS magnifying lens, so that the fluorescein patterns and lens movement can be observed. The magnification is less than the slit-lamp but there is a better overall view. If an ultraviolet filter is incorporated in the lens material a fluorescein pattern is not visible with a lamp, but can still be assessed using the cobalt filter on the slit-lamp.

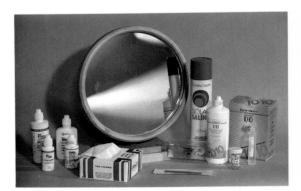

Figure 5.5   Equipment for teaching includes the patient's lenses, suitable solutions, tissues and a mirror

Equipment for teaching

For teaching, the patient's contact lenses, tissues, a starter pack of solutions and an appropriate container are required (Figure 5.5). A flat mirror placed on the table or an upright one on an adjustable stand is required. Most patients find a flat mirror, which should not have built-up edges, easier to use, some find a magnifying mirror more helpful.

Written instructions must be given to the patient. These are important as they ensure that all the important points relating to the care and handling of lenses are brought to the patients attention. They also act as a reminder, when the patient has returned home, and gives them confidence in the early days of lens wear. They should include how to insert and remove a lens by normal methods and in an emergency, details of how to care for the particular type of lens and instructions of when, where and how to seek urgent advice. A copy of suggested instructions is included in the chapters on fitting each type of lens.

Lens inspection and verification

All new lenses should be checked to ensure they are correct and that they are not damaged. Assessment of soft lenses is more difficult, and less accurate than for other types of lenses and requires special, expensive equipment, manufacturers will check lenses if requested. It is useful to measure and record the parameters of any lens which has been prescribed elsewhere. This should be done at the first visit so that, in the event of a lost lens, a new one can be supplied. Most of the essential lens parameters can be measured with simple equipment.

Radiuscope (Figure 5.6)

This uses the Drysdale principle to measure the BOZR of rigid lenses, which states that if an object is placed at the centre of curvature of a concave mirror, the image formed is real, inverted and the same size as the object and is situated at the centre of curvature. The clean lens is placed, concave surface upwards, on a holder containing distilled water, beneath a microscope. The water eliminates reflections from the anterior lens surface. The radiuscope is then adjusted until the upper or lower mires of the instrument are in focus, depending on the type of instrument. The scale is adjusted to zero and the microscope focused until the second set of mires are in sharp focus. The scale reading records the BOZR in hundredths of a millimetre. The radiuscope is more accurate than the keratometer (see below) but it is an extra expense.

The radiuscope may be used to measure the centre thickness of a lens. A flat plate is placed on the lens mount and focused by the microscope, the dial gauge is set to zero. The contact lens is placed concave side up on the flat plate and the

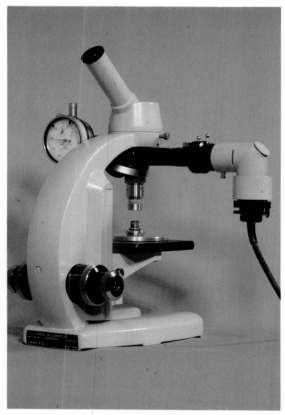

Figure 5.6 Radiuscope

microscope again focused. This reading is the lens thickness (Dickens, 1980).

Warpage can be seen when the radiuscope mires do not all focus simultaneously.

Keratometer

The BOZR of rigid lenses may also be measured by various devices that can be attached to the keratometer. The majority are mounts which hold the lens in the vertical plane by means of surface tension, a device of this type is available with the Canon autokeratometer. The contact lens acts as the surface of a concave mirror and measurements are taken in the same way as for an eye. The Con-ta-Chek (Figure 5.7) is a device, with a lens mount, which holds the lens in the horizontal plane and a mirror, above, is angled at 45° to the optical axis of the instrument. The reflection in the mirror acts as the image from which the keratometer mires are reflected.

This method of measuring the BOZR is less accurate than the radiuscope but it is convenient and less expensive, as standard equipment is used. Warpage can be detected from the keratometry readings.

Band magnifier (Figure 5.8)

A ×10 band magnifier has a graticule against which rigid lenses can be held manually and the BOZD and the OD can be measured directly. It

may also be used to assess the width of one or more PCs, providing that the transitions are sufficiently distinct to be seen. Well blended junctions will not have any definite demarcations. Lens edges can also be inspected using this instrument.

Tapered slot or V-gauge (Figure 5.8)

The lens is placed into the wide end of a V-shaped groove, concave side downwards, which is tilted so that the lens slides gently along the slot until it is stopped by the narrowing of the groove. The diameter is measured on the scale.

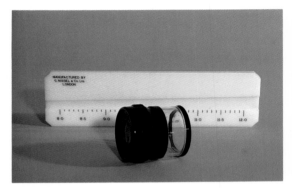

Figure 5.8   V-gauge and measuring magnifier

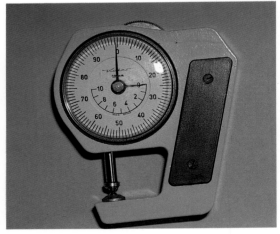

Figure 5.9   Hand-held thickness gauge (Ciba Vision)

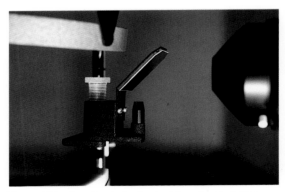

Figure 5.7   Con-Ta-chek attached to a keratometer

Thickness gauge (Figure 5.9)

A spring loaded thickness gauge is used. The lens must be carefully centred to obtain an accurate reading. The gauge most often used is an industrial one and care must be taken to release the spring gently or the lens may be damaged. A better instrument is a hand held gauge like the one marketed by Ciba Vision in which the release of the spring is controlled by a wheel. Centre and edge thickness can be measured (Dickins, 1980).

Slit-lamp

The shape of the lens edge is very important for comfort (Figure 5.10). It should be well-rounded with an edge thickness of 0.08–0.12 mm. Too thick and it is felt by the lid margins, too thin and it will be sharp and similarly uncomfortable. The lens should be inspected for any splits, rough areas and manufacturing marks.

The multiple curves on rigid lenses result in junctions which must be blended if the lens is to be comfortable. Blends may be observed by holding the lens directly beneath a fluorescent tube, without a diffuser, and examining its reflec-

tion in the lens (Figure 5.11). Alternatively the slit-lamp may be used. Junctions are too sharp if they are clearly visible. The slit-lamp, or a hand loupe, may be used to inspect engraving on a lens, as some trial lenses have their parameters engraved on them and some soft lenses have engraved reference numbers.

Soft inspection magnifier (Figure 5.12)

Soft lenses are very difficult to examine without expensive equipment. The soft lens analyser measures the BOZR of these lenses when the lens is

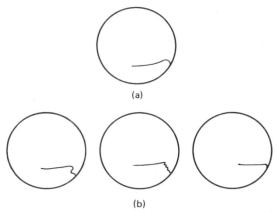

Figure 5.11 Examination of blends, (a) well blended lens and (b) inadequate blending

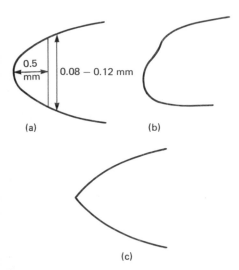

Figure 5.10 Diagram to show lens edge, (a) satisfactory well rounded edge, (b) irregular edge and (c) edge too sharp

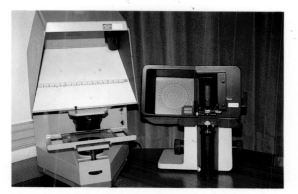

Figure 5.12 Inspection magnifier and projection focimeter

placed in saline in a wet cell. The radius can be compared with a series of hemispheres of known radius. The image of the lens is projected on to the template. If the lens vaults the template it is too steep and if there is apical touch it is too flat. The correct fit is found when the lens curvature exactly parallels the template. It is possible to use an overlaid scale to measure the CT, BOZD and width of the PC With soft lens inspection magnifiers the lens surface can be examined for damage and deposits, and the lens edge may be seen.

A simpler set of plastic templates has been used. The lens is placed on the model, if there is a bubble beneath the lens it is too steep, if the edge of the lens lifts away from the template the lens is too flat. This method is less accurate as the lens is not in saline.

Focimeter

The power of a contact lens can be measured using a standard focimeter with a smaller aperture stop. The lens must be placed against the stop of the focimeter and the back vertex power (BVP) is measured if the convex surface of the lens is towards the observer, the front vertex power (FVP) is measured if the concave surface is towards the observer. The advantage of recording the BVP is that lens thickness may be altered

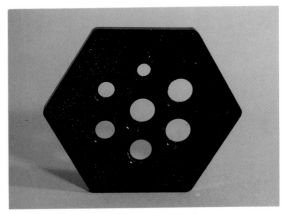

Figure 5.13 Contact lens adaptor for focimeter

without the power of the lens being affected. However the shape of the mount on most focimeters makes it difficult to remove the lens from the instrument if it is placed with its concave surface away from the observer. Either power may be used but it is important to inform the manufacturer which is being used and to ascertain from the manufacturer which parameter is used for his lenses, as there may be a significant difference between the two in the higher powers.

Rigid lenses can be measured by placing them in an adaptor (Figure 5.13) so that they are held against the stop. The reduced aperture increases the accuracy of the reading on an instrument that was designed for large spectacle lenses. The power of a soft lens may be measured by blotting the lens dry with lint-free tissue and placing it on the lens stop. An upright focimeter is best and readings need to be taken quickly or alterations will occur as the lens dries. Devices for measuring the power of lenses in wet cells are available.

With these parameters recorded it is possible to order a lens which is similar in all essentials to the original and a new lens can be evaluated.

References

ATKINSON, T. and KERR, C. (1987) The Kelvin Equalens design. *Optician*, January 2, 20–29

COTRAN, P. and MILLER, D. (1987) An adaptation of the Topcon slit-lamp for photokeratoscopy. *The CLAO Journal*, **13**, 277–279

DICKINS, R. (1980) Hard lens verification procedures. In *Contact Lenses*, 2nd edition, Volume 1, (eds J. Stone and A. Phillips), Butterworths, London and Boston p.295

PHILLIPS, A. (1980) Corneal lens fitting. In *Contact Lenses*, 2nd edn, Volume 1, (eds J. Stone and A. Phillips), Butterworths, London and Boston, pp. 265–275

PORT, M. (1985) The Canon Auto-keratometer K1. *Journal of the British Contact Lens Association*, **8**, 79–85

STEIN, H. and SLATT, B. (1984) Keratoconus. In *Fitting Guide for Rigid and Soft Contact Lenses, a practical approach*, 2nd edn, The C.V. Mosby Company, St Louis and Toronto, pp. 280–282

STONE, J. and FRANCIS, J.L. (1980) Practical optics of contact lenses and aspects of contact lens design. In *Contact Lenses*, 2nd edn, Volume 1, (eds J. Stone and A. Phillips), Butterworths, London and Boston. pp. 91–140

6

The initial visit and choice of lens

The wide variety of contact lenses which are now available makes contact lens wear possible for most patients. In order to select the most appropriate lens a full history and examination are required.

lens and the care system which were used may influence the choice of any subsequent lens. When possible it is useful to obtain the details of any previous lenses from the prescriber.

History

A complete ophthalmic history is taken which should include any systemic or ocular conditions which may influence contact lens wear, (see Chapter 1) and the reasons the patient wants contact lenses, so that the most suitable type of lens may be selected. Many patients have preconceived ideas about the type of lens they want to wear, based on recommendations from other lens wearers, advertisements or previous lens wearing experience. Successful wear may be more easily achieved if their wishes can be met, but if this is not practical the reasons for choosing another type of lens should be explained.

The strongly motivated patient will wear lenses more successfully than one who is inadequately motivated as they overcome the adaptation symptoms more readily and comply with proper lens maintenance. Patient motivation may include improved cosmetic appearance and better vision. Some patients are extremely apprehensive about wearing contact lenses, and may need to be considered psychologically unsuited to lens wear. It is essential when fitting children that they have understanding parents.

When there is a history of previous lens wear the problems which were encountered, the type of

Examination

A full ophthalmic examination and an accurate refraction should be done. Any refractive astigmatism should be compared with the corneal astigmatic keratometry readings (see Chapter 5). Residual astigmatism may require toric rigid or soft lenses (see Chapter 10). The features of the ocular examination which are particularly relevant to contact lens wear include:

Eyelids

The under surface of the lids should be smooth and regular so that there is adequate resurfacing of the cornea with tear film and should be examined for papillae and follicles. It is difficult to fit large lenses when the palpebral aperture is small, and a small lens may cause discomfort with a wide palpebral aperture because the contact lens is not covered by the upper lid. Ptosis may reduce lens movement and affect tear film exchange, and loose lids make it difficult to fit lenses using lid attachment techniques. The position and tension of the lower lid is important when lenses are stabilized by truncation or prism ballast and for fitting bifocal lenses (see Chapter 10).

The lid margins should be examined for trichiasis, blepharitis, entropion and ectropion. The openings of the meibomian glands may have blocked ducts or accumulated secretion. Any lid pathology should be treated before contact lenses are worn.

The blink rate should be assessed because patients with a reduced blink rate (normal is 16 per minute) may have difficulty wearing contact lenses. The completeness of each blink is also important as incomplete blinking may result in corneal drying, and three and nine o'clock staining (see Chapter 7).

Pupils

The size, shape, situation and reaction to light are recorded. Pupil measurements are necessary when cosmetic lenses are to be worn and if lenses are to be fitted without using trial lenses. An eccentric pupil may require a larger lens with a larger optic zone. The pupil diameter may be measured, in a dim light:

1. using an ophthalmoscope with a +10.0 D lens in the aperture and a millimetre rule;
2. with a graticule in the eyepiece of the slit-lamp; or
3. by measuring the pupil with a clear plastic scale from which metric circle templates have been cut.

The same methods can be used to measure the horizontal visible iris diameter (HVID) for calculation of the total diameter of a lens or the diameter of the iris of a cosmetic lens.

Conjunctiva

Any abnormality including pingueculae, scars and pterygia are noted, as patients may notice these for the first time when they are inserting their lenses, and assume they have been caused by the lenses. A large soft lens may ride up over a pterygium to produce astigmatism and instability of the lens. In this case smaller soft lenses, or RGP corneal lenses are preferable.

Active corneal and conjunctival disease must be treated before wearing lenses. Repeated trauma by rigid lenses to thin, conjunctival drainage blebs carries a serious risk of possible intraocular infection. Blebs, other than drainage blebs, should be removed if possible, before a lens is fitted.

Tear film

The tear film meniscus above the lower lid margin should be adequate and the tear film itself should be clean and free of mucus and debris. Fluorescein instilled in the eye will only fluoresce if there is sufficient tear film. The quality and quantity of the tear film can be estimated using Schirmers Test, which may show a marked abscence of tear film, and also the BUT (see Chapter 2). Soft lenses lose water on a dry eye, and the absolute decrease in water content is greater for high water content lenses than low water content lenses (Efron *et al.*, 1987). This should be taken into consideration when the marginally dry eye is fitted with a lens, as an RGP lens may be more suitable. Pathologically dry eyes may benefit from a therapeutic soft contact lens with copious rewetting drops.

Cornea

On slit-lamp examination using diffuse illumination, look for any evidence of keratoconus, keratoglobus, scarring or previous surgery. Focal illumination will show opacities and infiltrates and sclerotic scatter technique may reveal scars, ghost vessels and oedema. Retroillumination may show microcysts, blood vessels, bedewing and endothelial deposits. Specular reflection can be used to examine the epithelium for irregularities and the endothelium for dark areas indicating cell loss.

Inspect the cornea for dry spots, epithelial erosions and ulcers using fluorescein. Any abnormalities found before fitting with a lens should be recorded.

Corneal sensation is assessed (see Chapter 2) and keratometry readings are taken.

Choice of lens

The most appropriate type of lens for the patient must now be selected.

Indications for PMMA lenses

1. Patients who require very clear vision may prefer PMMA lenses which give more consistent vision than soft lenses. They are also effective in high astigmatism, without requiring a toric lens.
2. They are durable and do not break as easily as some RGP lenses. Lenticular lenses are less fragile and are better for aphakia with a heavy handed patient.
3. They are the least expensive lenses to buy and maintain.
4. The elderly often find them easier to handle than soft lenses and they may be removed with a suction holder if manual removal is too difficult.
5. There is less problem with deposit formation than with RGP or soft lenses.

Contra-indications to PMMA lenses

1. PMMA lenses may not be suitable for intermittent wear as tolerance is lost fairly rapidly.
2. They are less comfortable and require a longer adaptation period, and so are less satisfactory in the inadequately motivated patient.
3. They tend to be lost more readily than soft lenses, particularly in contact sports. Should a PMMA or RGP lens fall, being light it will tend to float sideways, and not drop straight downwards as does the heavier soft lens.
4. Dust under the lens may be a major problem at any time but particularly in dusty occupations and conditions, when soft lenses would be better.
5. PMMA lenses can cause definite endothelial changes after many years of use. This is most important in young patients, but not so important in elderly aphakics.

Indications for RGP lenses

1. Patients needing clear vision are usually best fitted with RGP lenses. If there is more than 1–1.5 DC of corneal astigmatism a low RGP lens should be used e.g. XL20 or CAB as they are less liable to flex on the eye.

2. Where PMMA lenses have resulted in discomfort, corneal oedema from hypoxia and endothelial changes.
3. When soft lenses are associated with papillary conjunctivitis or solution sensitivity reactions.
4. Patients with corneal warping from PMMA lenses may be fitted with RGP lenses to the same prescription, without having to stop lens wear, while the cornea is recovering.
5. RGP lenses can be larger than PMMA lenses which makes the lens fit more stable.
6. High *Dk* lenses may be used for extended wear.

Contra-indications to RGP wear

1. The lenses are more expensive than PMMA lenses to buy and maintain.
2. Deposit formation occurs more often and may make protein removing treatment necessary.
3. They are more fragile than PMMA lenses.

Indications for soft lenses

1. Soft lenses have been very popular with the general public as they are more comfortable to wear, cause fewer adaptation symptoms and can be worn intermittently.
2. They are more stable on the eye than corneal lenses, and are useful for sports wear.
3. Young children may tolerate a soft lens more readily than a PMMA or RGP lens.
4. They are useful in dusty surroundings.

Contra-indications for soft lenses

1. They have an average life-span of only 18 months to 2 years.
2. They are prone to deposit formation and discolouration and they can absorb air borne toxic substances such as aerosol sprays, perfume, cooking and chemical fumes and smoke.
3. Soft lenses will not usually correct more than 1 DC of astigmatism but will correct more than this if made thicker, at the expense of oxygen transmission.
4. Very thin and high water content lenses tend to be difficult to handle. If the lens is allowed to dry on the finger for a few seconds it will become more rigid, and be easier to manage.

Extended wear lenses

Three types of lens are in use for extended wear, high water content soft lenses, thin lower water content soft lenses and high *Dk* RGP lenses (see Chapter 9). These lenses are useful for those patients who cannot handle a lens because of age or infirmity. However the incidence of problems including the risk of serious corneal infection is higher than with other types of lenses and may progress rapidly under a contact lens. These lenses are therefore only suitable for fitting under close supervision and patients must be told to seek help urgently, the same day, from an ophthalmologist, if the eye is red, painful or has reduced vision. These patients will need to be prepared to attend regularly, at never more than three-month intervals. Poor attenders are not suitable for these lenses and they must be contacted if they fail to keep an appointment. If the patient cannot continue to attend, the lens should be removed, which may need a domicilary visit. Patients wearing these lenses should be told to inform medical and nursing staff about the lens if they are admitted to hospital.

Contact lens wearers should also have up-to-date spectacles, as they may be needed if contact lens wear is contra-indicated for a period, or if the patient wishes to remove their lenses in the evening or when they wake at night.

The patient should be warned that during the adaptation period there may be discomfort, watering and photophobia with some redness but that these will reduce as tolerance improves.

The full financial implications must be discussed. This involves the cost of the lenses, the necessary consultations for their fitting and proper aftercare together with the cost of solutions and the replacement of lost or damaged lenses.

By the end of the consultation the patient should have a clear idea of the type of lens selected, why and how they will care for it, what it will cost and how frequently they need to attend.

References

EFRON, N., BRENNAN, N.A., BRUCE, A.S., DULDIG, D., RUSSO, N. (1987) Dehydration of hydrogel lenses during normal wear. *CLAO Journal*, **13**, 152–155

Further reading

JONES, L. (1988) The use of high water content lenses on a daily wear basis. *British Contact Lens Association: Scientific meetings report*, 26–31

7

Rigid corneal contact lens fitting

Fitting PMMA lenses

A satisfactory PMMA contact lens should provide good visual acuity, be comfortable to wear and should not cause ocular problems. There are many different fitting techniques for these lenses but this chapter aims to provide the basic guidelines.

Principles of fitting PMMA lenses

1. The design, movement and overall size of the lens should ensure an adequate supply of oxygen to the cornea.
2. The lens should not interfere with the pattern of blinking.
3. The optic zone should be centred over the visual axis. Lenses are centred on the eye by the elastic forces associated with the meniscus which forms at the lens edge (Mackie, 1973). If the meniscus breaks below the lens can drop.

Fitting philosophies

There are many methods of fitting a lens; some depend on the overall size of the lens, others on central thickness but the most important feature is the relationship of the posterior lens surface to the cornea.

Alignment fit

Lenses are fitted 'on alignment' when the posterior curve (BOZR) parallels the curve of the cornea. For an average, spherical cornea and a lens

with a BOZD of 7.0 mm the keratometer reading may be ordered (Mandell, 1981). If the BOZD is increased the lens will be made steeper (see below) and apex clear.

Apex clear

These lenses are fitted so that they are slightly steeper than the flattest K-reading and vault the cornea. The lens of first choice would be halfway between the mean and flattest K-reading. As a general rule lenses are fitted slightly flatter than the mean K-reading if there is less than 1.50 D of astigmatism and steeper if there is more astigmatism. Corneas with more than 4.0 D of astigmatism may need a toric lens (see Chapter 10) but it is often possible to fit a highly astigmatic cornea with a spherical back surface PMMA or low Dk gas-permeable lens.

Lens–lid attachment technique

This method of fitting lenses was described by Korb and Korb (1970) to improve tear flow and so reduce the risk of corneal hypoxia. The lens should have the front surface of the peripheral carrier parallel to the back surface, or even slightly negative i.e. a negative carrier (Figure 7.1). This results in an increase in bulk at the periphery of the lens, which together with the minus flange allows the upper lid to grip the lens, so that it moves with the lid on blinking. A modified version of this technique has been found to be successful for correcting the position of low-riding plus lenses (Phillips, 1980). The lens needs to be drawn to scale to give the necessary lens parameters to the laboratory (Mackie, 1973). The

Persecon E Minus Carrier lens (Ciba Vision) is an RGP lens designed for lid attachment.

There is no one correct fitting philosophy but it is preferable to use the alignment technique for the majority of cases, modifying it when the occasion demands.

Contact lenses may be fitted with or without trial lenses.

Fitting without trial lenses

Photokeratoscope

Computer analysis of the photograph obtained by this method (see Chapter 5) does not provide information about the behaviour of the lens on the eye. The effect of the overall size of the lens, the degree of centration and the effect of the lids and blinking are only apparent when the prescription lens is placed on the eye.

Hartstein's method

This technique is based on measurement of K-readings, corneal diameter and the diameter of the

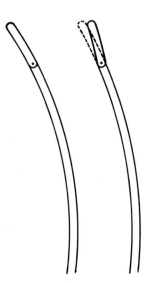

Figure 7.1   Diagram to show the 'idealogical hinge' in a negative peripheral carrier for lid attachment techniques (by kind permission of Ian Mackie)

semi-dilated pupil. The power is calculated from the spectacle refraction, with allowance made for back vertex distance (Hartstein, 1968).

LD+2 method

The total lens diameter is made 2.0 mm larger than the longest diameter of the corneal cap, as measured with the topogometer (Sampson, Soper and Girard, 1964). The photokeratoscope method is the only one which can be recommended, as it takes into account the peripheral curves of the cornea.

Fitting with trial lenses

Selecting the first trial lens

Select a trial lens, with a suitable BOZR, according to the fitting philosophy and the K-readings, from the fitting set. The lens should have a total diameter (TD) appropriate to the size of the palpebral aperture and horizontal visible iris diameter (HVID). Small corneas and palpebral apertures require smaller lenses, larger lenses may be needed for lens–lid attachment. The lens power is based on the spectacle refraction, adjusted for back vertex distance if there is more than 4.0 DS in the trial frame. The spectacle prescription is converted to the minus cylinder form and the cylinder ignored. The trial lens nearest to the spherical power is chosen. The lens should have an optic zone (OZ) large enough to cover the semidilated pupil (see Chapter 5).

Assessment of the fit

With the patient looking straight ahead the selected trial lens, wetted with wetting solution, is placed on the index or middle finger of the appropriate hand, concave side uppermost. The middle, or ring finger of the same hand holds the lower lid down, and the upper lid is held up firmly by the thumb of the other hand, to prevent a reflex blink (Figure 7.2). The lens is touched lightly onto the cornea and the lower lid released, before gently releasing the upper lid. If the upper lid is released first it may eject the lens from the eye without the lower lid to prevent it. The lens fit is now examined using the low power on the slit-lamp.

Lens position A lens should lie centred on the cornea, or slightly above, with the edge of the lens beneath the upper lid, if the lid attachment technique is used. The position of the lens should be noted and its movement with blinking observed. Lenses may ride high or low and be displaced temporally or nasally. A new wearer is liable to have orbicularis spasm, and a drop of local anaesthetic will help to relieve the spasm and watering, and aid the assessment of the contact lens fit. It is useful to use a drop of local anaesthetic before placing a lens on the eye if the patients previous response to eversion of the upper lid indicates a tendency to orbicularis spasm.

Lens movement Lens movement is essential, with PMMA lenses, for the tear pump to function and 1.0–2.0 mm of movement is acceptable. A lens which does not move is too tight and must be changed or corneal oedema may ensue. The optic zone of the lens should cover the pupil in all normal eye movements. A lens which touches or crosses the limbus is uncomfortable, and produces inadequate venting under the lens. A lens which moves excessively will also be uncomfortable, give unsatisfactory vision and may move from the cornea and out of the eye.

Optic zone Flare is the reflection of light caused by the prismatic effect of the non-optical part of the lens. Flare and ghost image occur when the

back optic zone diameter (BOZD) is too small and does not cover the semidilated pupil. It is often noticed by car drivers at night. A large BOZD may also be needed for patients with broad iridectomies. Altering the BOZD will affect the fit of the lens. Increasing the BOZD increases the sag value and steepens the fit of the lens, whilst reducing it will flatten the lens fit (Figure 7.3).

Total diameter (TD) The TD of the lens is assessed in relation to the size of the palpebral aperture, the cornea and any pterygia, sutures or surgical blebs. A lens may need to be smaller to avoid trauma to a thin bleb which may become infected and cause endophthalmitis.

Fluorescein patterns In order to see the lens–cornea relationship clearly a small quantity of fluorescein 2% is placed on the conjunctiva above the lens, with a fine glass rod. Too much dye with a watery eye makes the fit difficult to assess, and a glass rod controls the amount of glass used, without irritating the eye as much as a fluorescein impregnated paper strip. An irritated eye will cause copious tears which pool below, tending to pull the lens down.

The patient is asked to open and completely close the eyes gently several times to distribute the dye throughout the tear film and beneath the lens. The tear film is now examined with the blue filter on the slit-lamp or with an ultraviolet light, so that it fluoresces, and the fluorescein pattern is visible.

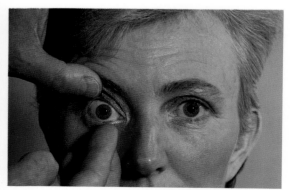

Figure 7.2 Clinician placing a contact lens on the patient's eye

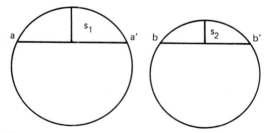

Figure 7.3 Diagram to show the effect of altering the BOZD on the fit of the lens. If the BOZD is reduced from aa' to bb' the sagittal depth is reduced from s_1 to s_2 and there is less 'vaulting' of the cornea by the lens, which is effectively made flatter. Increasing the BOZD will increase the sagittal height and the lens fit will be steeper.

1. *Alignment fit* This shows an even, thin layer of fluorescein beneath the OZ (Figure 7.4). An adequate edge lift is seen as a thicker, deeper green band of fluorescein under the flatter peripheral curves.
2. *Flat fit* The fluorescein is absent from the areas of touch, which may be central, or peripheral if the lens positions off centre (Figure 7.5).
3. *Steep fit* Dye will pool centrally, often with a circular, surrounding area of touch, with one or more bubbles beneath the lens. This fit must be avoided as it will lead to negative pressure under the lens and consequent corneal oedema (Figure 7.6).
4. *Corneal astigmatism* This will produce a toroidal, oval or band-shaped area of touch or clearance, depending on whether the fit is flat or apex clear centrally, with an abscence of dye where there is corneal touch (Figure 7.7, 7.8, 7.9).
5. *Edge lift* The edge lift of the lens and the tear film thickness can be estimated with fluorescein (Figure 7.10). Insufficient edge lift is one cause for an arcuate corneal stain.

If any of the lens parameters seem incorrect the lens is changed for another trial lens until a satisfactory fit is achieved.

Power

With a well fitting trial lens on the eye, an over refraction is done. When the patient is being

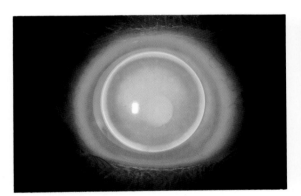

Figure 7.4   Alignment fit lens

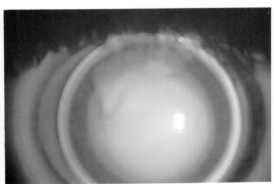

Figure 7.6   Tight fitting rigid lens with pooled stain centrally and peripheral ring of touch

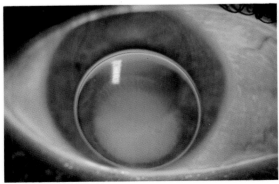

Figure 7.5   Loose fit with dropping lens – note apical touch and pooling of stain below

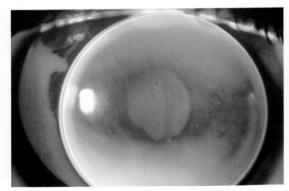

Figure 7.7   Astigmatic fit with central touch

refracted it is important that they blink gently and completely, to keep the lens clean and ensure the vision is stable. A correctly fitting lens should produce stable vision.

A residual refractive error may occur with rigid lenses when the K-readings and the refraction are dissimilar, and may need a toric lens (see Chapter 10).

To remove a rigid lens from the eye, pull the lower lid sideways, so that it is taut against the globe, which prevents the lens from going under the lower lid. The thumb of the other hand brings the upper lid margin down and under the lens, which is ejected from the eye, and caught between the thumb and finger (Figure 7.11).

Ordering the lens

The prescription should include the name of the laboratory, the patient, the material to be used, in this case PMMA, and the eye for which the lens is intended. All diameters, radii and powers must be stated with instructions detailing special data if these are not the same as the manufacturers trial lens set. The lens power must be clearly marked as BVP or FVP. The FVP is preferable as the lens is easier to manage on the focimeter with its concave surface towards you. In addition the following should be specified:

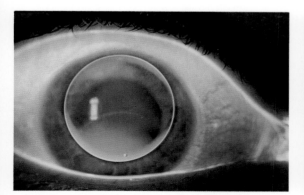

Figure 7.8   Astigmatic fit with central clearance

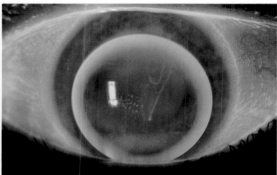

Figure 7.10   Foreign body stain and marked edge lift

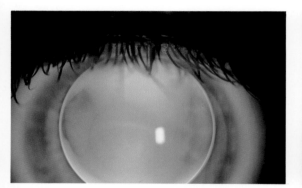

Figure 7.9   Astigmatic fit with high riding lens

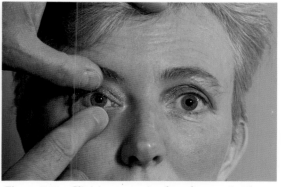

Figure 7.11   Clinician removing lens from patient's eye

Centre thickness

A thin lens is usually more comfortable than a thick one provided there is enough material to make a good edge but thin lenses are liable to warp and break. It is easier to manufacture a thicker lens and so the centre thickness should be stipulated and not left to the manufacturer. For a table of suggested average centre thicknesses see Appendix 2.

Blends

The junctions between one curve and the next will be sharp, and cause discomfort, unless they are blended (see Chapter 1). Heavy blending results in all the curves merging into one another and produces a lens which is almost continuously aspheric. Heavy blends appear at first to be the most desirable but can affect the fit of the lens. When light or medium blends are ordered further blending is possible if arcuate staining occurs.

Tints

Lenses are made of tinted material as an aid to locating them on the eye so that they may be found more easily when they are dropped and, less commonly, for cosmetic purposes. The most usual colour is light neutral grey, as this affects colour vision least, but a wide range and depth of colours are available in the grey, blue, green and brown ranges in PMMA. It is a help to have trial sets tinted in different colours so that it is easier to identify the different sets.

The final prescription for a tri-curve lens should look like this:

BOZR (BOZD)/ FBPR (FBPZD)/ SBPR (TD)
POWER
Tint, Blend, CT
where BOZR = Back optic zone radius
      BOZD = Back optic zone diameter
      FBPR = First back peripheral radius
      FBPZD = First back peripheral zone diameter
      SBPR = Second back peripheral radius
      TD = Total diameter
      CT = Centre thickness

It is important, when several clinicians work together, to have a standard procedure for recording lens prescriptions in the patients' records. These must be kept up to date by deleting any prescriptions which have been changed.

A correctly fitting lens centralizes well, has adequate movement on blinking, an even tear film under the lens and a satisfactory edge lift.

Fitting rigid gas-permeable lenses

Rigid gas-permeable (RGP) lenses are the most recent development in contact lens technology. They are often fitted as the lens of first choice, but are also indicated when corneal hypoxia occurs in PMMA wearers and when there are preservative hypersensitivity or toxicity problems in soft lens wearers. They are less likely to cause oedema, are more comfortable and require a shorter adaptation period than PMMA lenses, but are more prone to deposit formation. They are also more flexible, particularly those with high Dk values, and are less able to correct higher amounts of astigmatism unless the centre thickness is increased, or the lens changed for one with a lower Dk. The material is more fragile than PMMA and lenticular, high plus lenses may break at the junction of the optic and the carrier. RGP lenses give better visual acuity, will correct more astigmatism than soft lenses and are less prone to deposit formation and last longer.

There are five types of RGP lenses (see Chapter 3) and these can be divided into two groups, those with Dk values of less than 50, and those over 50 which are referred to as high Dk lenses. The latter can be suitable for extended wear and are dealt with in Chapter 10. Although the lower Dk lenses may be fitted using PMMA trial sets, the high Dk lenses should be fitted with trial lenses of the same material because of their greater flexure on the eye. The Boston Equalens, has an ultraviolet filter incorporated in the material. These lenses will not show a fluorescein pattern with ultraviolet light, but it can be seen using the cobalt filter on the slit-lamp.

Low Dk value lenses

The fitting technique for most RGP lenses is similar to that for PMMA lenses. The lens is fitted

on alignment, using fluorescein to assess the fit. Because of the oxygen permeability of the material, oxygen reaches the cornea through the lens as well as via the tear pump, and lenses can be larger than an equivalent PMMA lens. This produces better stability and centration and permits a large optic zone, which gives better vision. RGP lenses can be ordered thicker than a comparable PMMA lens, to reduce flexing and to correct more corneal astigmatism. The increased thickness should not reduce oxygen transmissability to the extent that the advantage of the *Dk* value is lost.

Silicone elastomer lenses

Silicone elastomer lenses are fitted near to the corneal diameter and 0.1 mm flatter than the flattest K-reading. They are almost impossible to remove from the eye by the pinching technique used for soft lenses and it is better to use the index fingers of each hand on the margins of the upper and lower lids to apply pressure to the edges of the lens.

Teaching the patient

The patient should be taught how to handle his lenses, which includes how to insert and remove the lens from the eye and how to care for it. The visit provides an opportunity for the patient to ask questions and it is important that sufficient time is available. The patient should not be allowed to take his lenses away until he can insert and remove them competently.

All the equipment needed should be available (see Chapter 5). The need for good hygiene and adherence to the instructions is explained and the consequences of failure are emphasized.

It should be explained to the patient that when inserting the lens the eye must be firmly held wide open, and the lids relaxed, as the blink reflex is very strong. Similarly on removing the lens the lids need to be held widely apart so that they lie above and below the lens. As the patient blinks, or moves the lids manually, the lid margins will pass under the lens edge and eject the lens from the eye.

The following notes are given to the patient at the time of the teaching session.

Notes for corneal lens wearers

Your cornea is like a transparent watch glass in front of the coloured part of your eye. It is living tissue and requires oxygen to maintain its transparency. The oxygen cannot come from the blood vessels as in other tissues, but oxygen in the air dissolves in the tear film from which it is taken up by the cells of the corneal surface. Unless there is an adequate change of oxygenated tear film under your contact lens, the cornea will suffer from lack of oxygen which will cause swelling of the surface cells of the cornea. This swelling will produce irritation of the eye, causing the blood vessels of the white of the eye to dilate, so that the eye appears red. If the irritation is marked, swelling of the eyelids may occur. Acute irritation of the eye tends to cause excessive watering, but chronic irritation and dryness tend to cause increased secretion of sticky mucus.

About your contact lenses

Hard corneal contact lenses are made of a plastic material (Perspex) and may easily become scratched, chipped or broken. Rigid gas permeable lenses are made from a mixture of materials to allow oxygen transmission through the lens. Being slightly softer they are even more easily scratched and broken, and should be handled with greater care. Take particular care when picking up a lens from a hard surface. Never bend or squeeze the lenses when handling them. **The lens for the right eye is marked with a small DOT near its edge, or engraved with an 'R'.**

Storage of lenses

Corneal contact lenses should be kept wet (hydrated) all the time, and never allowed to get dry. When wet they are much less likely to become scratched, and mucus is prevented from drying on the lens surface. When not being worn the lenses should be kept wet in antiseptic soaking solution in the container provided. Always clean them after wear before putting them in the case.

Cleaning procedure

1. Before placing the lens on the eye the hands should be washed with soap, such as Simple Soap, which does not contain cream or scent. Disinfectant hand solutions should also be avoided.
2. Handle the lenses, one at a time to lessen the risk of mixing the lenses.
3. Place the lens on the palm of the hand, concave (cup) side uppermost and fill with one or two drops of *cleaning solution*.
4. Massage both sides of the lens gently between the finger and thumb.

5. Always rinse off traces of the cleaning solution with rinsing/soaking solutions or sterile N-saline.
6. Check that the lens is clean by holding it up to the light.
7. Store the lens in the *soaking solution*.
8. Rinse the lens, when it is removed from storage, with rinsing/soaking solution or N-saline and fill the lens with *wetting solution* before inserting the lens.

Placing the lens on the eye (Figure 7.12)

1. Place the lens, concave side uppermost, on the tip of the index finger.
2. With head held straight, look directly into a small mirror in the middle of a white towel or large size paper tissue, with both eyes wide open.
3. Hold up the top eyelid and lashes with the middle finger of the other hand.
4. Use the bent middle finger of the hand holding the lens to pull the lower lid down.
5. Keep the eyes still by looking straight ahead into the mirror with the *other eye* and gently touch the lens onto the cornea.
6. Release the lower lid first and then slowly release the upper lid.
7. Check the vision to make sure the lens is on the cornea.
8. There are alternative methods for lens placement, one of which is to hold the lids apart with two fingers of one hand and place the lens on the cornea with the index finger of the other hand.

Recentring the lens

A lens may be left on the white of the eye without causing any harm, even if it is left there while sleeping.

If the lens is displaced below the cornea it may be recentred by looking into a mirror and using the lower lid margin to nudge the lens back on to the cornea. Both lids should be used if the lens is to the side. If the lens is under the upper lid, keep your head up and look right down, then lift the upper lid as high as possible and nudge the lens down on to the cornea. Never press the lens on to the white of the eye as this will tend to make the lens more adherent.

Lens removal

1. Sit close to a table.
2. Open the eyes really wide and place a finger vertically at the outer corner between the eyelids. Pull the lids tightly sideways and slightly upwards and a quick gentle blink should eject the lens from the eye or bring it to the eyelashes from where it can be removed (Figure 7.13).
3. Alternatively the index and middle finger of one hand are used on the upper and lower lids to eject the lens from the eye with a scissor-like action (Figure 7.14).
4. The middle fingers of both hands may be used; with the lower lid held taut with one middle finger, and the other finger to work the upper lid margin under the lens to eject it from the eye (Figure 7.15).
5. In case of any difficulty the lens may also be removed by holding the lids apart and splashing water into the eye–or using an eye bath.

Blinking

'Flick' blinking, so that the upper eyelid comes only halfway down over the lens, merely causes an irritation of the upper eyelid margin on the edge of the lens. *Correct blinking* entails looking straight ahead and completely closing both eyes together, just as though closing

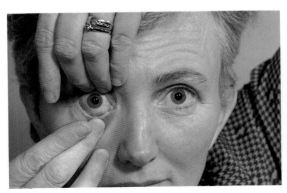

Figure 7.12   Patient – inserting lens

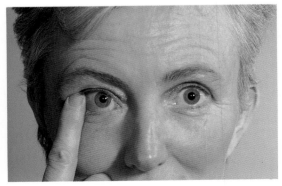

Figure 7.13   Patient – removing lens with one finger

the eyes to sleep, and then opening them wide again. It is most important never to squeeze the eyes closed when wearing lenses, as this will tend to press the lens on the cornea and cause irritation. Immediately after placing the lenses on your eyes, a few gentle blinks will make them comfortable more quickly. It is most important when blinking that you gently and completely close your eyes. If you are not having any problems you are blinking enough but if you are having problems you need to make sure you are blinking correctly and also blink more.

Correct blinking has the following objectives:
1. To wipe a fresh film of tears over the whole eye.
2. To cause a gentle movement and 'pumping action' of the lens on the cornea, ensuring a good tear flow under the lens so that the cornea receives an adequate oxygen supply.
3. To keep the front surface of the lens clean and free from mucus by the wiping action of the eyelids over the whole lens. If the lens surface becomes coated

with mucus, the upper lid will tend to stick to the lens, instead of gliding over its surface, causing irritation.
4. To acclimatize the eyelid margins to the presence of the lens which is the main cause of initial discomfort.

Wearing schedule and after-care

Wearing time should be increased gradually and consistently. The following is a recommended wearing schedule:

2–4 hours for the first day, increasing by an extra 1 or 2 hours every day until all day wear is achieved.

If more convenient, the lenses may be worn for two to three periods a day with short breaks in between (a minimum of two hours) until all day wear is reached.

You should always be wearing the lenses when you come for a check visit, and the longer you have been wearing the lenses the more valuable the check.

If the lenses have not been worn at all for several days, the wearing time should be cut in half initially, and then increased by 2–4 hours a day. You will be advised on how often you should attend for check visits; initially this will depend on your progress. Eventually a check once a year is recommended even though you may not be having any problems. At these visits the condition of the lenses themselves will be examined.

General points:

1. Do not rub your eyes when wearing contact lenses.
2. Never sleep with a lens on your cornea, unless you have been told it is safe to do so.
3. It is inadvisable to swim or sunbathe when wearing contact lenses, in case you lose the lenses or fall asleep in them.
4. Do not drive wearing contact lenses until you are satisfied that your vision is adequate. This is particularly important at night when you may notice haloes or streamers round lights.
5. Do not use hair and other sprays unless you keep your eyes closed until the air is clear, as the lacquer can damage your lenses.
6. If an eye is painful do not wear the lens again until the eye has been completely comfortable for at least 24 hours.
7. Always seek medical advice should the eye remain consistently red and/or painful.

When first beginning to wear contact lenses you may find:

1. Some blurring of vision with spectacles after removal of your lenses. This may last from a few minutes to an hour or so, and may require a change of lens.
2. A greater sensitivity to bright light which is commonly caused by inadequate blinking. Polaroid sun-

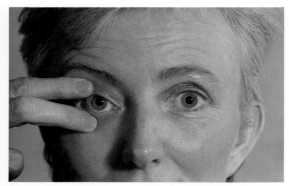

Figure 7.14 Patient – removing lens with two fingers

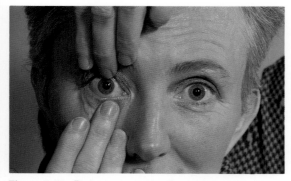

Figure 7.15 Patient – removing lens using top and bottom lids

glasses may be worn outdoors as they will reduce the reflected glare from below.
3. Discomfort in a warm, dry atmosphere when the tear film evaporates more quickly, and particularly in a smokey atmosphere.
4. Discomfort when reading, driving, watching TV or a film is due to an increased tendency to stare and insufficient, incorrect blinking.
5. An excessive watering of the eyes, or mucus on the lenses. Sudden lid movements may then dislodge the lens from the cornea or even out of the eye.

Should you experience any of these problems they should all become less as you become used to your contact lenses.

Rigid lens follow-up

The follow-up examination is similar to the initial examination.

History

A careful history is taken of the patients progress and symptoms from the time lens wear started. It is important to determine which problems are contact lens related and which are not.

Wearing time

The amount of time the lenses are worn each day, the wearing time (WT) gives an idea of how well the patient is managing, as well as the amount of tolerance acquired. Patients who are having difficulty handling their lenses, or who are apprehensive, wear their lenses for short periods only. The WT is recorded as, for example WT=3(8). The first figure indicates the number of hours the lens has been worn prior to that examination and the figure in brackets is the length of time, in hours, for which the lens is normally worn each day.

Blurred vision (Table 7.1)

This may vary between alteration in quality of vision, with no actual reduction in the recordable acuity, to markedly diminished visual acuity.

Corneal oedema is the most important cause of blurred vision associated with contact lens wear (Figure 7.16). The vision is reported as reduced or hazy, and in severe cases haloes may be seen. Hypoxia is the main cause of oedema and the lens must either be exchanged for an RGP lens or the PMMA lens must be refitted or fenestrated to improve venting.

The power of the lens may be incorrect due to an error by the clinician or the manufacturer. The lens should be checked for power on the focimeter, and the BOZR should be checked with a radiuscope or keratometer, as this may also affect the power. If the error lies with the manufacturer the lens is returned for a new one. If the lens is incorrect then a new lens to the amended power is ordered. Alterations up to $\pm 0.5\,\mathrm{D}$ to the original lens are possible but it is better to order a new lens.

Residual astigmatism is another cause of blurred vision (see Chapter 10).

Lenses may be inserted in the wrong eye. Lenses are usually marked with a single dot or 'R' for the right eye. It is a simple matter to identify the lens

Table 7.1 Causes of reduced visual acuity associated with contact lenses

Normal change in refractive error
Inaccurate power of lens
Switched lenses
Residual astigmatism
Warped lens
Dirty lens
Deposits on soft or RGP lenses
Stromal oedema
Watering eye
Poor centering

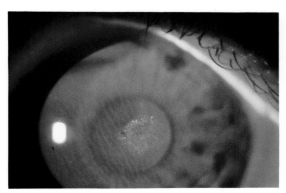

Figure 7.16   PMMA lenses – hypoxic keratitis

and reinsert it in the correct eye. However it is sometimes found that neither lens is marked. Identification then relies on checking the lenses for power, BOZR and TD and comparing these with the known prescription. If the lenses were prescribed elsewhere it may be possible to identify them if there is a significant difference in the refraction of the two eyes.

Excessive watering reduces the visual acuity. It is often present during the adaptation period and should gradually improve. Persistent watering has other origins (see below).

Dirty and scratched lenses cause blurred vision (Figure 7.17). Cleaning and reinserting the lenses should produce an immediate, marked improvement in vision. RGP lenses which have not been surface treated respond well to Boston Cleaner (Polymer Technology) and greasing of lenses requires intensive cleaning with a cleaner such as Miraflow (Ciba Vision Contactasol). Tear film substitutes should be used frequently and meibomian gland and other lid disease (Figure 7.18) should be treated. Any lens with scratches should be polished, or renewed if the scratches are deep.

If a lens is not centred, because of an unsatisfactory fit or excessive movement, the vision will blur intermittently.

A badly fitted or warped lens will result in hazy vision.

Spectacle blur is a condition which occurs when rigid lenses are exchanged for spectacles, perhaps at the end of the working day. The patient has blurred vision due to corneal oedema and/or 'warping'. The corneal warping is more likely to occur with high amounts of corneal astigmatism and a spherical back curve lens. The refraction is changed by the corneal thickening and altered curvature and punctate staining may occur. The resulting corneal irregularity is concealed by the precorneal tear film when the lens is on the eye, but becomes apparent when spectacles are worn. Spectacle blur should be improved by a change to RGP lenses.

Burning

A burning sensation occurring as soon as the lens is placed on the eye may be due to a dirty or damaged lens, a foreign body or mucus under the lens, or sensitivity to the wetting solution. The lens may also be inserted, mistakenly, with a non-isotonic cleaning solution, instead of a wetting solution. Cleaning solution may also cause burning if the lens has not been rinsed after cleaning and before insertion. This may cause a punctate keratitis which can take days if not weeks to resolve.

If burning is reported after several hours wear the problem is likely to be a tight fit of the lens and reduced tear flow, leading to corneal oedema. The fit of the lens should be altered or an RGP lens used instead.

Pain and discomfort

Severe pain associated with a marked reduction in vision occurs in the so-called 'over wear' or 3 a.m. syndrome. There is a history of the patient having

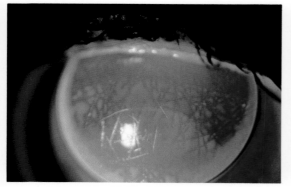

Figure 7.17 Scratches on rigid lens

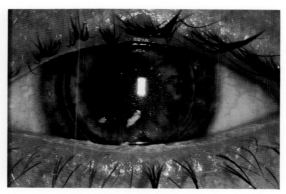

Figure 7.18 Blepharo-conjunctivitis with rigid lens

worn the lenses all day, often for a longer period than previously, but with no apparent problem when they remove their lenses. Typically they are woken by pain, during the early hours of the morning, which may be so severe that they seek urgent treatment. Local anaesthetic drops are needed to relieve the pain in order to examine the eyes. There is lid swelling, conjunctival and ciliary injection and confluent, central punctate keratitis. Treatment involves a cycloplegic (guttae cyclopentolate 1%) to relieve the ciliary spasm, analgesics for pain and a tranquillizer or hypnotic to help them sleep. The eye must be padded after putting in antibiotic ointment. If both eyes are affected the possibility of using a therapeutic soft lens, with intensive antibiotics, should be considered for one eye. The syndrome is due to dry eyes, incorrect and insufficient blinking, a tight fit or dry atmosphere. PMMA lenses should be changed for RGP lenses of adequate gas permeability.

Discomfort may be experienced as one of the adaptive symptoms (see below) or may be due to lid problems (Figure 7.18) such as lenses which are too large or too small for the palpebral aperture so the lid margins are irritated by the lens.

Lens edges which are too thick or badly shaped are a common cause of discomfort.

A dirty lens is uncomfortable and wet stored lenses are more comfortable on insertion than those stored dry.

To improve the corneal oxygenation, when corneal oedema occurs with PMMA lenses, one to three holes 0.3 mm in diameter may be drilled through the lens. These fenestration holes can cause a problem if they are badly finished or when mucus is trapped and dries in the hole (Figure 7.19). It is important that the back surface of the fenestration is well countersunk and polished. The front surface should be only lightly countersunk or it may produce a 'waterfall' effect down the front of the lens which can interfere with vision.

Flare

Flare can occur, particularly when driving at night. If it is due to too small an optic zone the symptoms will be relieved when the pupils constrict with a bright light. This effect is easily demonstrated if the test is carried out in a dark room. Flare can also be due to a badly centring lens so the patient is looking, intermittently, through the unfocused periphery of the lens. In this instance the flare is more variable and is improved by stabilizing the lens. In both cases a larger BOZD on an RGP lens should solve the problem.

Photophobia

Photophobia is common as part of the adaptation symptoms and the patient can be told that it should gradually reduce. However, if the problem persists, other causes such as corneal oedema, too large a lens or three and nine o'clock staining should be sought. Improved oxygen transmission can be obtained by changing to an RGP lens or a smaller PMMA lens. Dryness of the eye should be treated with lubricant eyedrops such as SnoTears (Smith and Nephew) or Liquifilm Tears (Allergan).

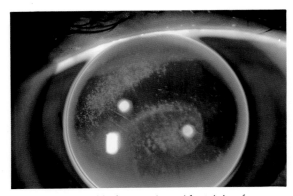

Figure 7.19 Double fenestration with staining from dried mucus in the holes

Redness and watering

If these persist after the initial period reduced blinking or tear flow may be the cause. Corneal oedema is associated with red, watery eyes as are lens related problems such as poor edges and transitions. If hypoxia is the cause the lens should be changed to an RGP lens or one with a higher *Dk* value. If the lens is the cause it should be modified.

Lens awareness

An uncomfortable lens is usually caused by edges which are too thick or badly finished and this results in increased lens movement which aggravates the problem further.

Lens loss

This may occur when lenses are too small or too flat. Small lenses tend to be mobile and may move off the cornea or be ejected from the eye. Patients who report the loss of a lens should be examined carefully. There are many instances of lenses being retrieved from the upper fornix and of lenses embedded in the tarsal plate (Talbot, 1986) for long periods. The lid should be doubly everted to examine the palpebral conjunctiva and, if a drop of topical anaesthetic is applied, the upper fornix can be explored with a thin, sterile glass rod (Figure 7.20). The impact of the rod on any retained contact lens can be felt and heard and the lens can be swept from under the top lid.

Difficulty with close work

This usually occurs during the adaptation period. Myopes no longer have the benefit of the prismatic effect of their spectacles and notice the greater need to accommodate. The majority adapt well in a few weeks.

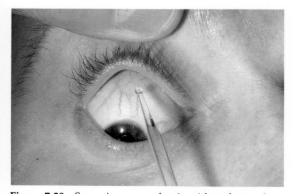

Figure 7.20 Sweeping upper fornix with a glass rod

Handling problems

Difficulties in inserting and removing the lenses often respond to further teaching. If removal remains difficult, and the patient can identify the lens on the eye, then they may be given a suction holder for removing the lens. It is important that the patient is sure that it is placed on the lens and not the cornea to avoid corneal trauma. Solid suction devices are preferable to hollow ones. They are wetted and touched lightly on the lens to remove it gently from the eye. The lens is removed from the holder by pinching behind the suction cup. Handling problems which occur from loss of dexterity, sensation or deformity may mean the patient needs an extended wear lens.

Many of the symptoms to which the patient may refer on the first follow-up visit are so-called 'adaptive symptoms'. These occur in the early stages of wear when lens tolerance and handling skills have not developed. They include watering, photophobia, discomfort, foreign body sensation and lens awareness. The patient should be warned about these symptoms and assured that they will gradually reduce.

Examination

The longer the patient has been wearing the lenses the more informative the findings.

Overall appearance

Watering or redness may be due either to lens related factors or possible pathology.

Altered blinking may be caused by an interpalpebral lens producing irritation of the lens margins. A larger lens with thinner edges which is covered by the upper lid will cause less discomfort and should produce normal blinking. Attention to correct and adequate blinking will increase corneal wetting, clean the lens, reduce redness and increase comfort.

A mild ptosis can occur in one or both eyes, early or later, from contact lens wear. It may be associated with a defective or badly fitting lens, or a problem under the upper lid or of the cornea. A thinner RGP lens with a lid attachment fit may

help, or it may be necessary to refit the patient with soft lenses.

Visual acuity

The visual acuity with contact lenses is checked with an over refraction. If an alteration in power is required up to ±0.5 DS, it is possible to alter the existing lens but it is preferable to order a new lens. Causes of reduced vision associated with PMMA or RGP lenses are listed in Table 7.1.

Slit-lamp examination using white light

Lens position and movement

The position of the lens is noted, particularly with reference to movement on normal blinking.

High riding lenses This often occurs with high minus lenses whose thick peripheral edges produce lid attachment. Other causes are with-the-rule astigmatism (plus cylinder at 90°), or a flat fitting lens. Patients with updrawn pupils or broad iridectomies benefit from a high riding lens, and are fitted with a lid attachment lens in order to centre the optic zone near to the visual axis. An excessively high riding lens may cause visual problems and requires a larger lens with a larger optic zone. A prism ballast of up to 1.5Δ may help to bring the lens down as will a thinner plus carrier by reducing the lens–lid attachment.

Low riding lenses This occurs with thick, heavy, high plus lenses. The lens may be too small or too flat. It may drop jerkily because of with-the-rule astigmatism, or from tight lids and is often seen early in contact lens wear due to orbicularis spasm.
   A dropping lens can be made larger or steeper but, preferably, a high minus carrier should produce lid attachment.
   Altering the BOZR of a rigid lens, to make the lens steeper or flatter, will produce a change of power. The effective power of a lens depends on the curvature of the front and back optics and a plus lens which is made steeper will produce an increased plus tear film under the lens from the increased sagittal height and require less plus power to produce the same vision. Similarly a minus lens which is made with a steeper BOZR will need more minus power (Appendix 5).

Horizontal displacement A lens may become displaced either nasally or temporally after the blink. This is usually associated with against the rule astigmatism, common in aphakia, or an eccentric corneal apical zone. Temporal displacement can usually be corrected by a toric peripheral curve on the lens (see Chapter 10). Alternatively a steeper lens or a larger OZ, which will increase the lens clearnace (sag value), can be used to stabilize the fit.

Lens movement A PMMA lens should move about 1.5–2.0 mm with the blink. An RGP lens may move less as it does not rely entirely on the tear pump to supply oxygen to the cornea. However a lens may sometimes de-centre or fall out of the eye, because of excessive movement. Lens movement should be examined in relation to the blink and in all positions of gaze. A lens which de-centres continuously at the lower limbus will be uncomfortable and may cause neovascularization. The lens edge should be inspected as a thick, or badly made edge, may be pushed down more by the upper lid. Stability can often be improved by making the lens larger.

Location of optic zone

The position of the OZ should be checked as discussed above.

Total diameter

Interpalpebral lenses tend to be uncomfortable and may be a cause of three and nine o'clock staining and Dellen. The TD may need to be increased to make the lens more stable, or reduced if the lens is likely to interfere with draining blebs, sutures or pterygia. If a bleb is large it may be possible to reduce its size surgically before a lens is fitted. Sutures should be removed as soon as possible after surgery. Reducing the diamter of a PMMA lens will increase lens mobility.

Lens fit

The fit of the lens is assessed as on the initial visit (see Chapter 6).

A tight lens will show minimal movement with the blink, with central pooling of the stain and peripheral touch impeding tear exchange. This can result in negative pressure under the lens making lens removal difficult and causing corneal oedema. The patient complains of blurred vision and a burning sensation. A tight lens can be caused by a lens which decentres, so that the OZ fits steeply onto a flatter area of peripheral cornea. The lens should be changed for a flatter one, with a larger BOZR.

A flat fitting lens is more mobile than an alignment fit lens. The lens may ride high if it is a high minus lens and low if it is a heavy, plus lens. There may be excess edge lift and corneal touch. A steeper lens with a smaller BOZR is required.

Corneal staining

Corneal staining with fluorescein has a variety of causes, many of which show typical stains.

A zig-zag or looped stain may be caused by a foreign body as it is moved by the up and down movement and rotation of the lens on blinking (Figure 7.21).

Wedge shaped areas of punctate stain occurring at three and nine o'clock (Figure 7.22) are the result of drying due to inadequate tear film. A lens with a thick edge may hold the lid away from the eye, so preventing normal tear film distribution and inducing abnormal blinking. If the condition is allowed to persist there may be thinning of the stroma to form a Dellen (Figure 7.23). Improved blinking, thinner edges and lubricant eye drops are all helpful.

Arcuate staining may occur above and below towards the corneal periphery as the result of a sharp lens edge or insufficient blending or transitions. Soaking solution may dry on the lens and if this is not carefully removed, before the lens is inserted, can cause similar staining. Single or double arcuate stains may occur with badly finished transitions (Figure 7.24).

Bubble impressions (Figure 7.25, 7.26) can be mistaken for punctate stains. They result from an air bubble which is trapped under the lens,

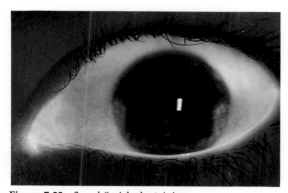

Figure 7.22   3 and 9 o'clock staining

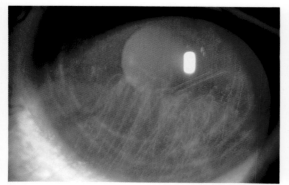

Figure 7.21   Foreign body stain – note vertical and rotary movement of lens with blinking

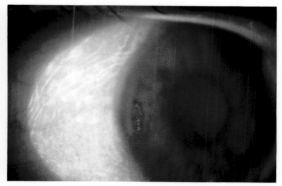

Figure 7.23   Dellen

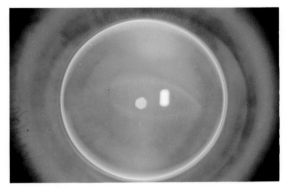

Figure 7.24   Central fenestration with double arcuate staining

breaking up into a series of small bubbles. These indent the corneal epithelium and fluorescein pools in the indentations. The indents are discrete, circular, variable in size and larger than punctate stains. The fluorescein rapidly washes away if the lens is removed.

A linear corneal stain can be caused by a scratch with a long fingernail during lens insertion or removal. Patients must be advised at the initial visit to keep their nails short, or to be careful.

Corneal dry areas may be seen when fluorescein is instilled (Figure 7.27).

Conjunctival staining may occur in dry eyes (Figure 7.28).

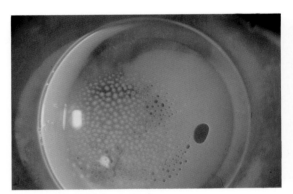

Figure 7.25   Bubbles under lens

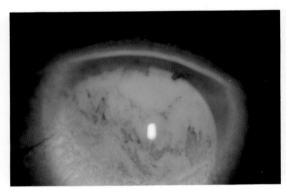

Figure 7.27   Cornea with dry areas

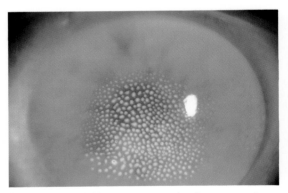

Figure 7.26   Bubble impressions after lens removal

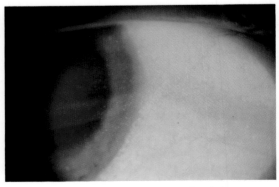

Figure 7.28   Dry eye with conjunctival staining

Corneal oedema

It is best seen with the lenses removed from the eye, using the sclerotic scatter technique (see Chapter 2), as an area of central epithelial oedema. It is due to insufficient venting and results in a reduced wearing time. The cause may be a tight lens, dry eyes or inadequate blinking. The staining caused by the oedema may vary from discrete to confluent punctate staining. The PMMA lens should be replaced by an RGP lens. If a PMMA lens is preferred, because of higher astigmatism, it can be fenestrated with one to three holes, 0.2–0.3 mm in diameter.

Corneal neovascularization

This can occur with large, thick, high-riding PMMA lenses and dropping lenses, both of which may cross the limbus and cause corneal hypoxia. In severe cases the patient must stop wearing the lens while the vessels regress, and they should then be fitted with middle *Dk*, RGP lenses.

Lens inspection

Lens integrity

It is important to ensure that the lens is undamaged by examining it with the slit-lamp or a band magnifier. Elderly patients with reduced sensation in their fingers, often wear lenses with damaged edges and may be unaware of this when wearing

the lens. Lenses may also develop cracks, and although the crack may not cause symptoms, a defect in the lens surface may collect mucus and debris. Such a lens should be replaced as soon as possible and the patient warned of the condition so that they will handle the lens very carefully.

Deposits (Figure 7.29)

On PMMA lenses these are likely to be due to cosmetics, particularly eyeliner and mascara. Patients should be warned not to use liner or khol inside the lash margin and to avoid mascara with 'lash-lengthening' fibres. Products should be water soluble so that they can be cleaned from the lens. Care should be taken to shut the eyes if aerosol hair sprays are used while the lenses are worn. If hairspray contaminates the lens surface it can be removed with ethyl ether.

Greasing of lenses and excessive mucus secretion are associated with deficient or altered tear film, lens scratches or lid margin disease (Figures 7.30, 7.31 and 7.32).

RGP lenses are more prone to protein and lipid and mucus deposit formation (Figure 7.32) than PMMA lenses and if this occurs protein removing enzyme tablets may be used, (see Chapter 4). Should hard dried mucus occur, particularly as a peripheral ring (Figure 7.33) the lens can be repolished.

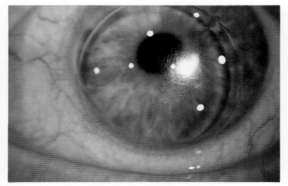

Figure 7.29 White paint spots on rigid lens

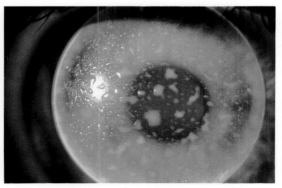

Figure 7.30 Grease on a rigid lens (meibomian secretion)

Scratches

Superficial scratches are common on PMMA and RGP lenses and the majority require no attention. Deeper scratches (Figure 7.34) may be polished off but there is a risk of lens distortion. If the scratches are deeper still the lens should be renewed.

Lens edge

The lens edge should be inspected using the slit-lamp or a profile analyser, and the blending of the transitions checked (Chapter 5).

Warping

If warping is suspected check the lens on the radiuscope or keratometer, when a warped lens will show astigmatic distortion of the mires, but a focimeter (lensometer) will give a spherical reading.

Refitting contact lenses

Any patient who has been fitted elsewhere should be treated as a new patient with regard to the refraction and K-readings. If the vision cannot be

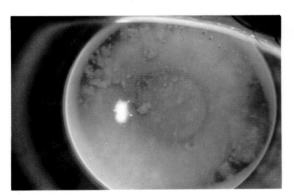

Figure 7.31   Clumps of mucus on a lens

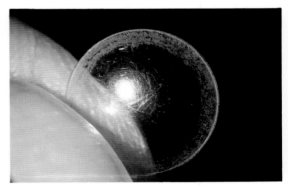

Figure 7.33   Peripheral ring deposit on RGP lens

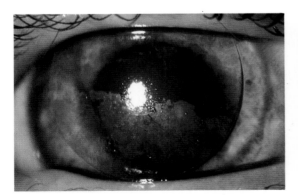

Figure 7.32   Dried mucus on RGP lens. The film is on the lower half of the lens showing that the patient is only 'flick' blinking.

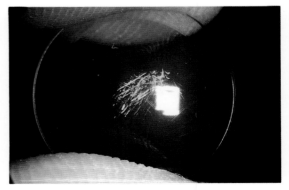

Figure 7.34   Central rigid lens scratches

corrected satisfactorily, or if the keratometer mires are blurred and misaligned, it is necessary to wait a few days before repeating them. Often, however the patient does not have any satisfactory spectacles and cannot manage without their contact lenses. In this case new lenses must be ordered (see below).

If the vision, with the present lens, is less than 6/6 but the fit is satisfactory, an over-refraction is done. If this improves the vision to 6/6 then a new lens is ordered with the same specifications but a new power. If the fit is satisfactory and the visual acuity is normal then the same lens may be reordered.

Evaluation of lenses fitted by others

History

This should include the daily wearing time and the total period for which lenses have been worn. It is useful to know what types of lenses have been tried and their problems. Details of the lens solutions which have been used may indicate possible causes for sensitivity reactions or lack of hygiene.

Examination

The visual acuity is recorded with contact lenses and with spectacles, if any. The conjunctivae are examined for sensitivity reactions, papillae or follicles, the cornea for oedema and staining and the lens assessed for fit.

Lens inspection

Examine the lenses for damage and warping. The state of the edges and the blends is noted and whether the correct lens is on the eye. Finally the lens BOZR, TD and power are measured and the lens details recorded.

Prescribing spectacles for occasional wear

Because of the problem of spectacle blur with PMMA lenses it is often difficult to achieve satisfactory vision with spectacles for the rigid contact lens wearer.

Various recommendations are made about the length of time for which contact lenses must be left out of the eye before an adequate refraction is obtained. If the patient has some spectacles, or if they can be driven to the consultation, see them early in the morning, not having worn their lenses that day. If this is not possible, then get them to remove their contact lenses on arrival, and refract them half an hour later. If satisfactory vision is obtained, and the patient only wishes to wear glasses in the evening, this should be satisfactory. An alternative solution is to refract one eye at a time. The patient should be warned that spectacles are unlikely to give as good vision as their contact lenses. There is less of a problem in providing glasses for RGP lens wearers although some difficulty may still occur. The complications of rigid contact lens wear are summarized in Table 7.2.

Corneal sensation is reduced when rigid contact lenses are worn. Cessation of wear results in a gradual return of corneal sensitivity over a period of weeks or months.

Changes in corneal curvature sometimes occur with PMMA lenses, which may be due to corneal oedema or moulding. If corneal moulding occurs RGP lenses may be prescribed, as an interim stage, before fitting soft lenses or the lenses should be left off the eyes until the parameters are stabilized.

Table 7.2 Corneal complications of rigid contact lens wear

Corneal staining	Corneal warpage
Arcuate or ring	Orthokeratology
3 and 9 o'clock	Hypoxic oedema
Foreign body	Overwear syndrome
Abrasion	Neovascularization
Corneal Dellen	Endothelial cell alteration
Lens induced	Infection
hypoaesthesia	Hypersensitivity reactions
Change in corneal	Giant papillary
curvature	conjunctivitis

Keratoconus has not been proved to be due to lens wear and this is unlikely (see Chapter 12).

Orthokeratology has been used to produce corneal flattening by fitting flat lenses but is rarely used now.

Hypersensitivity reactions are not often seen with rigid lenses. They are reactions to the care solutions and may be eliminated by prescribing solutions containing different preservatives or entirely preservative-free solutions e.g. hyrogen peroxide systems.

Giant papillary conjunctivitis associated with rigid lens wear is characterized by papillae appearing first near the lid margin. It is more common with RGP lenses, particularly those with protein deposits.

References

HARTSTEIN, J. (1968) *Questions and Answers on Contact Lens Practice*, C.V. Mosby Co., St Louis, pp. 99–102

KORB, D.R. and KORB, J.E. (1970) A new concept in contact lens design. *Journal of the American Optimetric Association*, **41**, 1023–1032

MACKIE, I.A. (1973) Design compensation in corneal lens fitting. In *Symposium on contact lenses: Transactions of the New Orleans Academy of Ophthalmology*, C.V. Mosby Co., St Louis, pp. 65–81

MANDELL, R.B. (1981) *Contact Lens Practice*, 3rd edn, Charles C. Thomas, Springfield, Illinois, pp. 168–178

PHILLIPS, A.J. (1980) Corneal lens fitting – fitting techniques. In *Contact Lenses*, Volume 1, 2nd edn, (eds J. Stone and A.J. Phillips), Butterworths, London and Boston, pp. 266–267

SAMPSON, W.G., SOPER, J.W., GIRARD, L.J. (1964) Designing the semi-finished lens. In *Corneal Contact Lenses* (ed. L.J. Girard), C.V. Mosby Co., St Louis, pp. 127–146

TALBOT, E.M. (1986) Upper eyelid chalazion or lost hard lens complications. *Journal of the British Contact Lens Association*, **9**, 88–89

Further reading

DIXON, J.M. (1964) Ocular changes due to contact lenses. *American Journal of Ophthalmology*, **58**, 424–443

RUBEN, M. (1967) Corneal changes in contact lens wear. *Transactions of the Ophthalmic Society of the United Kingdom*, **87**, 27-43

STONE, J. (1981) Designing hard lenses in the 1980s. *Journal of the British Contact Lens Association*, **4**, 130–137

8

Daily wear soft contact lenses

Many potential contact lens wearers have preconceived ideas that they would prefer soft lenses, owing to the extensive publicity that they have received. The possible problems of soft lenses have not been so well publicized, and these should be discussed with the patient.

Provided there are no definite contra-indications to the patient having soft lenses (see Chapter 6), and having decided to fit them with daily wear soft lenses, a choice has to be made from the many which are available. Most manufacturers make lenses to their standard specifications (Appendix 8, Table 8.2). Some of these manufacturers will make lenses outside their standard range, but at an increased cost, and a delay in availability. Some smaller manufacturers will make soft lenses to an individual prescription. Having found a dependable manufacturer, whose lenses and service are consistently reliable, it is best to stay with them as far as possible. Most clinicians however use two or three manufacturers to give them a range of different BOZRs, sizes, water contents and thicknesses.

there is minimal corneal astigmatism, and the patient is capable of handling a thin lens. Standard thickness lenses will correct more corneal astigmatism than thinner ones. It should never be necessary to use anaesthetic drops when fitting a soft lens, and never use fluorescein, which can be difficult to remove from the lens. A pHEMA lens of average standard thickness can be used as an initial example. Trial lenses are essential, and these usually have BOZRs in 0.20 mm differences. Start with a lens diameter about 1–2 mm larger than the corneal diameter (HVID) see Chapter 7. A 13.00 or 13.50 mm total diameter lens is suitable for most purposes, but a larger diameter may be necessary for a large cornea. Many manufacturers say 'fit the flattest lens you can, which is stable on the eye', but with no guidance as to where to start. Higher water content, and thinner lenses will cover a wider range of K readings, and are sometimes made in steep and flat fits only.

The Ciba Vision Weicon 38E and CE lenses are made with an elliptical back surface, which flattens gradually towards the periphery. This produces an even overal lens thickness, and a comfortable lens.

Daily wear lathed soft lens fitting

Following an accurate refraction, keratometry, and eye examination, the choice lies between a thin lens, or one of standard thickness. A basic requirement is a pHEMA lens fitting set of 38% water content, both as standard thickness, and as thin lenses, and in a range of BOZRs and overall diameters. A thin lens is preferable, provided

Table 8.1 Initial soft contact lens BOZR

Mean K reading (mm)	Initial BOZR for the lens diameters below added to mean K reading				
	13.0	13.5	14.0	14.5	15.0
7.00 to 7.49	0.60	0.80	1.00	1.20	1.40
7.50 to 7.89	0.50	0.70	0.90	1.10	1.30
7.90 to 8.29	0.40	0.60	0.80	1.00	1.20
8.30 to 8.70	0.30	0.50	0.70	0.90	1.10

The BOZR of a standard pHEMA initial lens may be assessed from Table 8.1. From the keratometer readings, and the lens diameter, the table gives the amount which must be added to the mean K reading, to give the BOZR of the lens. Thus a mean K reading of 7.80 and a 13.50 mm TD lens will need a BOZR of $7.80 + 0.70 = 8.50$ mm. If the value found lies between two BOZRs that are available from that manufacturer, always choose the flatter lens. The aim when fitting a soft lens is for it to give good stable vision, and be comfortable, without causing any corneal changes. Ideally the lens should be the flattest fit that is stable on the eye.

Before handling a soft lens, the hands should be thoroughly washed with Simple Soap, to avoid lens contamination with scented or cream soap, and particularly with disinfectant hand creams and solutions. The hands should be dried with a lint free, or paper towel. It is important that the patient sees this being done, as it stresses the importance of them doing the same, when handling their own lenses. Having decided on the BOZR and TD of the lens you need, choose a trial lens of these specifications, and as close as possible to the estimated spherical power required. Before opening the bottle containing the lens, it should be shaken gently to make sure the lens is mobile in the solution, and not adherent to the cap.

To remove the lens from the bottle, an ideal instrument is a sterile plastic ointment applicator which is individually packed. When removing the applicator from its envelope, do not touch the flattened end, which is used for removing the lens from the bottle (Figure 8.1). The front surface of the lens is put on the tip of the index or middle finger, having first made sure the lens is not inside out (Figure 8.17).

West German lenses (Ciba Vision and Wohlk) have lightly engraved (laser) numbers round the lens periphery (Figure 8.2), which can only be read correctly from the front surface of the lens. A hand loupe with a magnification of ×8 or more is usually required to read the numbers. The back surface of the lens which is to be placed on the cornea, should never be touched with the fingers. With the lens on the tip of the index finger, the upper lid is held up by the thumb of the other hand, and the lower lid held down by the middle

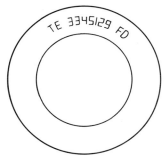

Figure 8.2 Laser engraved identification around periphery of soft lens (Courtesy of Ciba Vision)

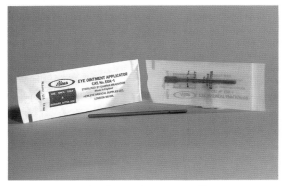

Figure 8.1 Sterile plastic ointment applicators

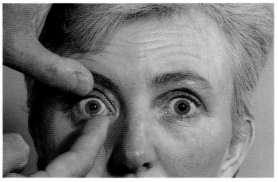

Figure 8.3 Placing soft lens on patient's eye with one finger

finger of the same hand. With the patient looking straight ahead with the other eye and at eye level, the lens is gently touched on to the cornea (Figure 8.3). It may be easier to place the lens on the middle finger, and to hold the lower lid down with the ring finger, as it is shorter. Some patients will tend to look upwards, or attempt to close the lids. Should this happen it may be easier to ask them to look downwards, and to touch the lens on the conjunctiva above the cornea. As the patient closes their eyes, the lens should move down onto the cornea. Some lenses, e.g. very thin lenses, are difficult to manage with this method, or the patient may tend to squeeze, and present only a small interpalpebral fissure. In these cases it may be easier to hold the lens by its front surface at the lower edge between the thumb and forefinger, (Figure 8.4) and place the upper edge up under the upper lid. When a patient has small deep-set eyes it may be easier to hold the lens as in last method, but pull the bottom lid away from the eye while the patient looks down, and then to place the lens well down behind the lower lid. Whichever method is used, the lower lid should always be released first, otherwise the upper lid may 'roll' the lens up and eject it from the eye. This is particularly likely to happen if the lens is too tight, when a bubble may have formed under the lens.

Examine the eye on the slit-lamp to check that:

1. The lens is on the cornea.
2. Part of the lens has not folded under at one edge.

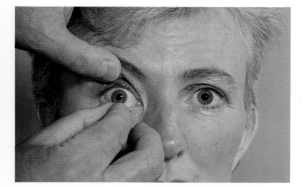

Figure 8.4 Holding soft lens between thumb and forefinger to place on patient's eye

3. There is no FB under the lens, e.g. mucus, mascara or an eyelash.
4. There is no bubble under the lens.

If the edge has rolled under or there is an FB under the lens, the lens should be removed, and its back surface sprayed with an aerosol of N-saline before replacing the lens on the eye. If there is a bubble under the lens, this can be removed by gentle massage over the upper lid with the eye closed, or by asking the patient to open and close the eye several times. An alternative method is to use the lower lid margin to push the lens up on the cornea, and then asking the patient to blink over the lens, which should express the bubble from under its lower edge.

At least 15 minutes should be allowed for the lenses to settle on the eye, so that the fit can be assessed for lens centration, and lens movement with eye movements and blinking.

Assessing the fit

Good fit

There should be good centration when looking straight ahead, and on looking upward the lens should drop slightly by 1–1.5 mm at most. With normal blinking the lens should move slightly, and then return to a central position. The reflex with the streak retinoscope will remain clear on blinking. With keratometry, there is no distortion of the mires before and after blinking.

Loose fit

There will be excessive movement of the lens on blinking, and with eye movements, particularly on looking upwards (Figure 8.5). If very loose, the lens may move completely off the cornea. The lens will not centre well, and there may be bubbles under the periphery of the lens. There may be localized lifting of the lens edge (Figure 8.6). The reflex with the streak retinoscope will be clear initially, and will blur after blinking, and then clear again. The keratometry mires will be clear at first, blur after a blink, and then clear again.

Tight fit

There is little or no movement of the lens on the eye on blinking, or with eye movements. There may be a bubble under the central area of the lens initially, and blanching of the conjunctival vessels under the edge of the lens. After a while there may be conjunctival indentation by the edge of the lens (Figure 8.7). The reflex in the streak retinoscope will be blurred initially, will clear after a blink and then go blurred again. The keratometry mires will be blurred initially, and clear when the lens is flattened by a blink. Should a lens fit be too loose or too tight, it should be changed for the appropriate tighter or looser lens.

To remove a soft lens from the eye, ask the patient to look up, slide the lens down on to the conjunctiva below, and pinch the lens off the eye between the thumb and forefinger (Figure 8.8). The new lens is allowed to settle before checking the fit again. There is a relationship between the TD and the BOZR of a soft lens, in order to keep the fit the same. If the TD is increased by 0.5 mm, the BOZR should be 0.2 mm flatter. If the TD is decreased by 0.5 mm, the BOZR should be 0.2 mm steeper. Thus a lens may be made a tighter fit by increasing the TD as well as by steepening the BOZR, and may be made a looser fit by reducing the TD, or flattening the BOZR.

The aim is to have a lens which centres well on

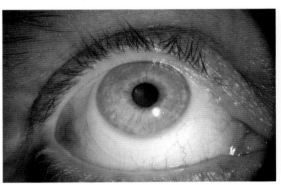

Figure 8.5   Excessive movement of soft lens on looking up

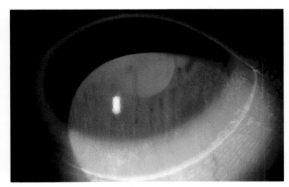

Figure 8.7   Tight fitting soft lens with fluorescein pooling in the conjunctival impression caused by the lens edge

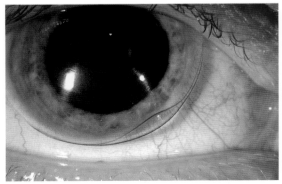

Figure 8.6   Loose fitting soft lens with edge lift (rucking up) below

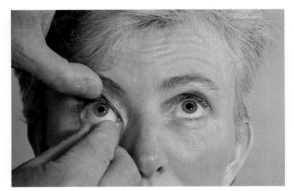

Figure 8.8   Removing a lens from patient's eye by pinching between thumb and forefinger

the cornea with full corneal coverage, and an equal overlap all the way round of 1 mm or more. While full corneal coverage is necessary, completely symmetrical lens centration is not essential. The lens should move slightly with eye movements, and with blinking. It cannot be stressed too often that soft lenses must never be fitted too tightly. Having ensured that the lens fit is satisfactory, a refraction is done over the lenses. If the patient is satisfied with a spherical over correction, the lenses can then be ordered. If there is residual astigmatism of 0.75 DC or over, and the patient is not satisfied with the vision, then toric soft lenses should be ordered, (see Chapter 10) or a change made to PMMA or RGP lenses.

When ordering the lenses from the manufacturer, it is only necessary to specify the BOZR, the TD and the power, e.g. 7.80 (13.50) −4.00 DS.

Fitting spun cast lenses

Fitting a spun cast lens such as the Bausch and Lomb Soflens the procedure is slightly different, as the FOZR is the same for all lenses in a particular series. The BOZR will vary with the power required, as this is the sum of the dioptric power of the front and back curves.

The Soflens is fitted by the 'First Fit Method', which is designed for obtaining the best fitting lens, with the minimum number of trial lenses.

1. Estimate refractive error, and correct it for back vertex distance.
2. Measure the horizontal visible iris diameter (HVID).
3. Select the power from the refraction.
4. If the HVID is 11.75 mm or less, choose a 13.5 mm TD lens. If the HVID is greater than 11.75 mm, choose a 14.5 mm TD lens.
5. From Appendix 8, Table A8.3 select a thin lens, e.g. U or O series, and place on patient's eye for up to 15 minutes.
6. Should the lens decentre and not completely cover the cornea, a large and/or thinner lens should be tried.
7. A well fitting lens should have full corneal coverage with good centring, some lens movement with blinking and eye movements, and acceptable comfort.

To order a Bausch and Lomb Soflens, it is only necessary to give the series number and the power, e.g. U3 −4.50 DS.

Instruction on the care and handling of soft lenses

The following are written instructions given to patients at the time of their teaching session, but see Chapter 4 for information on solutions used for lens care.

Instructions for the use of daily wear soft contact lenses

Soft contact lenses are made from hydrophilic (water loving) plastic, which has the ability to absorb water like a sponge. They can have different water contents, and daily wear soft contact lenses range from about 35–70 per cent water by weight. If allowed to dry, a lens will shrink, but if handled carefully and placed in the soaking solution, they will hydrate satisfactorily without being damaged. The lens must always be kept in a solution when not being worn. Cleanliness is most important when handling soft contact lenses. The hands should be washed thoroughly and dried with a lint free or paper towel. Try to avoid using hand creams, deodorants, after-shave lotions, and similar cosmetics prior to handling the lenses. Eye make-up should be applied after inserting the lenses. Long or sharp finger nails can damage a lens or your eye. Some lenses are engraved with numbering which aids lens recognition, but you may need a magnifying lens in order to read them.

Lens insertion

1. Wash, rinse and dry your hands thoroughly.
2. Remove lens from container, and shake off excess solution.
3. Check to ensure lens is not turned inside out. This may be done by flexing the lens between the thumb and forefinger, open side upwards. If the edges point inwards the lens is the correct way round – if not the edges will turn outwards. Alternatively check by the code numbers, if you have been told your particular lenses have them.
4. Place lens on top of index finger of dominant hand, and pull lower lid down with the middle finger of that hand.

5. Raise top lid with middle finger of other hand, making sure that both lids are pulled apart by the lashes.
6. Place lens on the eye, and after removing index finger release lower lid first (Figure 8.9).
7. Blink gently to centre the lens, and then check your vision to make sure the lens is on the cornea.
8. If the lens is below the cornea, it may be moved on to the cornea by light pressure on the lower lid from below the lens. If the lens is to either side of the eyes, look in the opposite direction, and use top and bottom lids to slide the lens on to the cornea. All these movements can be done when looking in the mirror. If the lens is under the upper lid it cannot be seen in the mirror. With the head erect, and slightly backwards, look down as far as possible, then lift the top lid up also as far as possible and move the lens down with the upper lid margin. The lens should slide down on to the cornea with gravity.

Lens removal

Method 1   Open eye wide and place appropriate index finger pointing upwards inside the outer corner of the eye, making sure your finger tip is on both lids at the same time. Pull lids tightly sideways towards the ear, and blink to eject the lens, and catch in other hand.

Method 2   Push the lower lid margin against the white of the eye with one index finger, and push the top lid also against the white of the eye with the other index finger. The lids must be open slightly wider than the diameter of the lens.
  Bringing the lids together should eject the lens.

Method 3   With the middle finger of dominant hand pull lower lid down. Looking straight ahead, place index finger on the lens and slide it downwards on to the white of the eye. Keep finger on lens, look upwards and pinch lens off the eye between thumb and forefinger (Figure 8.10). Should a lens be difficult to remove, try splashing the eye with saline solution or water.

Daily wear soft contact lens follow up

Suggested intervals for soft contact lens reviews are at one to two weeks, one month, three months and then six monthly from starting lens wear.
  The timing may need to be altered for convenience, or if problems arise such as a red, uncomfortable, or painful eye, or blurred vision. If any of these occur, the lens must be removed immediately, and advice sought from an ophthalmologist.
  Always attend wearing your lenses for a minimum of three hours whenever possible, provided there are no particular problems.
  Lens containers, any spare lenses, and spectacles should be brought to every visit. Soft contact lenses need to be removed to examine the eye properly, and lenses may need to be left for thorough cleaning.

  These instructions are given to patients to use at home, when they may have forgotten the verbal instructions given to them.

At a routine soft contact lens visit:

1. Ask what current or other problems have occurred since the last visit.

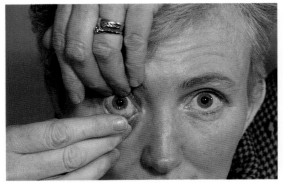

Figure 8.9   Patient placing soft lens on eye

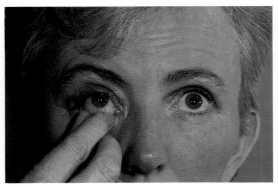

Figure 8.10   Patient removing soft lens from eye

2. Check the vision with soft contact lenses, including an over refraction, as a myope may be over corrected. It is important that the patient has arrived wearing their lenses. If no change is found record as VR plano–>6/6 with CL. An alteration of 0.50 DS or more may be changed if the patient wishes it. A power change should be altered and dated on the lens prescription in the notes. If a change is found check that the correct lens is on the eye, and that it is not inside out; this is when engraved numbered lenses are invaluable. Alteration of refraction can be caused by partially dehydrated lenses, and an increase in myopia may be caused by lens surface film and deposits. Thorough cleaning, or a new lens to the same prescription should restore the vision to normal.

3. Slit-lamp examination to check the lens for centration and movement, and any damage, surface film or deposits.

4. Remove lenses.

5. Slit-lamp examination of the lids, corneae, bulbar and palpebral conjunctiva. If fluorescein has been used, irrigate eyes with N-saline, and leave lenses out for 15 minutes if possible.

6. Examine lenses with the slit-lamp, a microscope, or a projection magnifier, for any defects, and to check the lens numbers when present.

7. If the vision in soft contact lenses has not been satisfactory, and cannot be improved, remove the lenses and check the vision with spectacles, as it may be a soft contact lens cause, and the vision can be improved to normal with spectacles.

8. Check the keratometry, tonometry, and corneal thickness and sensation whenever indicated.

9. It should be continually stressed to patients that soft contact lenses must be removed immediately should the eyes become red or painful and if there is any discharge or blurring of vision. Should any of these problems occur, an ophthalmologist must be consulted as soon as possible.

Complications of daily wear soft lenses

Lens complications

Lens damage

This may occur from faulty handling. Edge defects can result from the lens being caught in the lid of a lens container. Splits or tears can occur from long sharp finger nails, particularly when cleaning the lens or removing it from the eye or container (Figure 8.11). Higher water content and thinner lenses seem more prone to damage, and some patients tend to be 'accident prone' and 'heavy handed'. Lens dehydration and surface damage make the lens more likely to develop surface film and deposit formation. Surface damaged lenses can become contaminated with infective organisms, and are better replaced. However, lenses with edge defects such as small tears, or when small fragments are missing, can continue to be used so long as the lens is comfortable. The patient should be warned not to wear the lens if any symptoms of possible infection such as redness or discharge occur. Lenses can discolour, particularly to yellow and brown from the use of adrenaline (epinephrine) eye drops, and nicotine from smokers fingers (Figure 8.12). Ageing lenses have a tendency to go yellow and curl up, and are difficult to handle.

A rust spot or ring may occur on the surface of the lens, from an embedded particle of ferrous metal. This causes no problem unless it is in the visual axis, and can have the advantage of distinguishing one lens from the other (Figure 8.13).

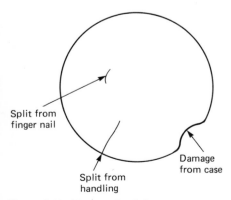

Split from finger nail

Split from handling

Damage from case

Figure 8.11 Damaged soft lens

Lens contamination with film and deposits

A common complication; as any soft contact lens which has been worn, if only for a few hours, may develop some surface film and deposits (Tripathi, Tripathi and Ruben, 1980). The incidence is increased with dry eye conditions, and by incorrect inadequate blinking (Figure 8.14). The lens surface must be kept clean and smooth, for good vision and comfortable wear.

Surface film may occur on both surfaces of the lens, but is chiefly on the front surface. When on the under surface it causes marked corneal irritation and a very uncomfortable lens (Figure 8.15). The lens must be thoroughly cleaned before being

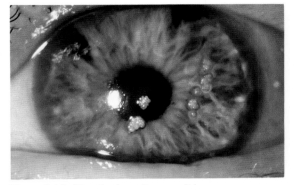

Figure 8.14   Protein deposits on soft lens

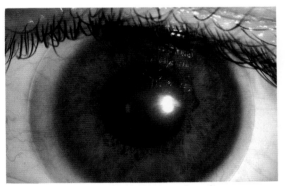

Figure 8.12   Brown soft lens from adrenaline (epinephrine) drops

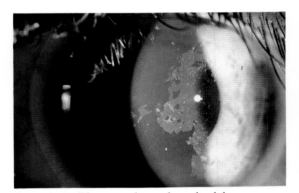

Figure 8.15   Film on under surface of soft lens

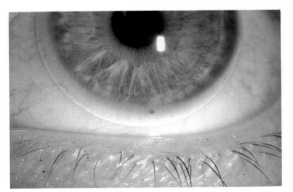

Figure 8.13   Small rust ring on soft lens at 6 o'clock periphery

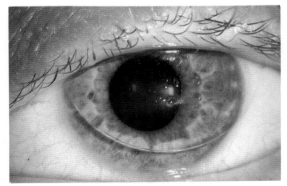

Figure 8.16   Soft lens central deposit – note lens being drawn upwards by upper lid

worn again. When deposits occur on the front of the lens, the lens may position high on the eye, and may even be lifted up under the upper lid out of view (Figure 8.16).

Surface film and deposits should be cleaned from the lens on removal from the eye, with a surfactant solution, before overnight soaking. A hypertonic saline solution which shrinks the lens, aids removal of contaminants from the inside and surface of the lens. Avoid cleaning solutions containing thiomersal, particularly when a hypersensitivity reaction has occurred. Even a small trace of thiomersal can trigger off a further and worse reaction. An enzyme protein remover can also be used every one or two weeks. Surface film and deposits are derived from lacrimal, mucous and meibomian secretions in the tear film, which contains lysozyme, albumin, globulin, lipids and calcium. A dry eye will concentrate these tear film constituents, which can form the surface film and deposits (Tripathi, Tripathi and Ruben, 1980).

Lenses with deposits require intensive cleaning with Liprofin or Monoclens. Preventive daily cleaners include hydrogen peroxide 3%, Softab (chlorine), Aerotab (halazone), Pliagel and Miraflow (see Chapter 4).

Lens absorption

Fumes, smoke, aerosol sprays, and the contents of eye drops and contact lens solutions may be absorbed by lenses. Some of these can have an allergic or toxic effect on the cornea and conjunctiva, but can usually be removed from the lens by intensive cleaning.

Inside out lenses

It can sometimes be difficult to tell whether a lens is inside out or not. If inside out, the patient may find the lens uncomfortable, and the vision poor or variable. To check a lens hold it between thumb and forefinger, open side upwards. If correct the edges turn inwards, and if inside out the edges will turn back on the fingers (Figure 8.17). Wohlk and Ciba Vision lenses can be distinguished by their numbers. The early engraved lenses had large deep and easily read engraving, but this often attracted protein deposits. Present laser engraving is lighter and smaller, which makes it more difficult to see, but much easier to keep clean.

Lens loss

Lenses lost from the eye are usually found, as the hydrated lens being heavy will tend to fall vertically. However, lenses may adhere to clothes, furniture and other objects. A lens can disappear under an upper lid particularly if it becomes folded, and can be difficult for the patient to locate. If a lens cannot be found on eversion of the upper lid, a drop of local anaesthetic in the eye will enable a fine glass rod to be swept under the upper lid to check whether the lens is still there. This saves the embarrassment of a lens reappearing subsequently, after you have told the patient that the lens is not in the eye.

Tight lens

A lens which moves adequately on the eye at the beginning of the day can become tight and relatively immobile by the end of the day from dehydration. This is more likely to happen in dry eyes, when blinking is incorrect and inadequate, and particularly from dry air conditioning, car heaters, prolonged reading and looking at computer screens. A tight immobile lens can produce conjunctival indentation by the lens edge (Figure 8.7). Debris can be trapped under the lens, and

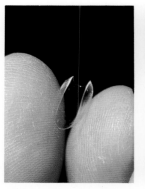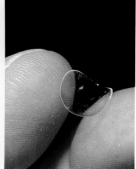

Figure 8.17 Soft lens correct way on left, and inside out on right. Note that an inside out lens turns its edges back onto the fingers.

epithelial oedema may occur from corneal hypoxia.

Reducing the TD, or a flatter BOZR will give a looser fit.

Loose lens

The lens will move excessively with eye movements and blinking, and may move off the cornea at times. There may be air bubbles under the lens periphery, with edge lift in places (Figure 8.6). The vision will be intermittently unclear and the lens uncomfortable. A larger TD, or a steeper BOZR will give a tighter fit.

Fungus on lenses

Fungus can grow on daily wear lenses, but is more common on extended wear lenses (Bernstein, 1973; Yamaguchi *et al.*, 1984). It is often seen on lenses which have been stored in unpreserved saline (Figures 8.18 and 8.19). Fungi are killed by 1 hour in hydrogen peroxide 3% and by thermal disinfection. An infected lens must be replaced.

Conjunctival complications

Chemical conjunctivitis

Substances absorbed by the soft lens, such as preservatives in contact lens solutions may cause a chemical conjunctivitis (Mondino *et al.*, 1982). An

example is benzalkonium chloride which can cause conjunctival hyperaemia and chemosis, as well as corneal changes. Inadequate rinsing after the use of enzyme preparations, and inadequate neutralization of hydrogen peroxide, can also produce the same effect (Stenson, 1986).

Infective conjunctivitis

If there is a red eye and discharge, the lens must be removed immediately, and the eye examined by an ophthalmologist. An acute bacterial infection may commonly be caused by *Staphylococcus aureus*, haemolytic streptococci, pneumococci, and the *Haemophilus* and *Proteus* species, usually with a purulent or muco-purulent discharge. Swabs are taken for culture and drug sensitivity; treatment is started with antibiotic drops, and changed if indicated by the laboratory report. Viral diseases include adeno-keratoconjunctivitis and inclusion conjunctivitis with a follicular conjunctivitis. Follicles are discrete aggregations of lymphoid tissue, commonest in the lower fornix and essentially avascular. Typically they are greyish white, round to oval, and 0.5–1.5 mm in diameter. Vessels surround, but do not enter a follicle.

Allergic conjunctivitis

This can occur from preservatives in the lens care solutions, or in any eye drops which are being used with the lenses. Symptoms include:

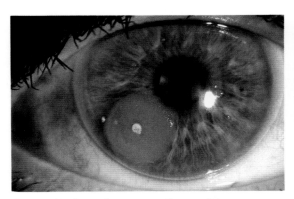

Figure 8.18   Large fungus growth on soft lens

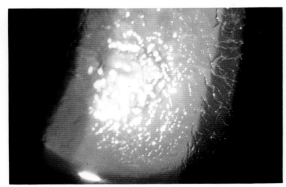

Figure 8.19   Fungus hyphae on soft lens (high magnification)

1. Itching.
2. Increased lacrimation and mucus secretion.
3. Conjunctival and limbal hyperaemia and chemosis.
4. Papillary and/or follicular response under the lids.

Protein film and deposits on the lens surfaces, particularly the front, are also thought to act as the antigen for the allergic reaction. Trantas's dots may occur at the limbal area (Meisler *et al.*, 1980). Treatment consists of thoroughly cleaning the lenses to remove the antigen, and stopping any drops or solutions which might be causing the allergy. A contaminated lens should be replaced with a new one. The lenses should then be cleaned on removal each night with a surfactant which does not contain any thiomersal or chlorhexidine preservative. The surfactant, and the disinfecting solutions subsequently used should also be preservative free.

Giant papillary conjunctivitis (GPC)

This condition was first reported by Spring in 1974, and was further investigated by Allansmith *et al.*, 1977; Mackie and Wright, 1978; Richmond and Allansmith, 1981; Price *et al.*, 1982; Donshik *et al.*, 1984 and Greiner, Fowler and Allansmith, 1984. Conjunctival papillae, particularly under the upper lids, are a common finding in any young patient, particularly teenagers. Their incidence and size can increase markedly in contact lens wearers, and are thought to occur in 1–5% of hard lens wearers and 10–15% of soft lens wearers (Greiner, Fowler and Allansmith, 1984). Symptoms include:

1. Itching.
2. Excessive mucous discharge.
3. Increased lens movement on the eye.
4. Blurred vision from lens film and deposit.
5. General discomfort when wearing the lenses.

The upper tarsal conjunctiva may be divided into three zones for purposes of description (Figure 8.20).

A soft contact lens is often displaced upwards from the cornea, by the upper lid which becomes attached to the lens by the tenacious sticky mucous discharge (Figure 8.21). The discharge coats the lens, often within minutes of inserting the lens, and produces blurred vision. Typically the conjunctival papillae occur under both upper lids, but can be unilateral. In soft lens wearers they tend to appear first in the area farthest away from the lid margin (Figure 8.22), and spread to include the whole upper lid surface, with a gradual increase in size. Initially the papillae of GPC were defined as larger than 1.00 mm but now includes papillae exceeding 0.33 mm in diameter (Greiner, Fowler and Allansmith, 1984). The papillae have the appearance of elevated cobblestones (Figure 8.23). Each papilla has a central fibrovascular core, with a central vessel which becomes a radiating collection of vessels on the surface of the papilla.

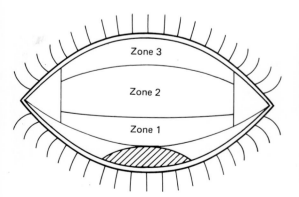

Figure 8.20 Upper palpebral conjunctiva divided into zones for descriptive purposes

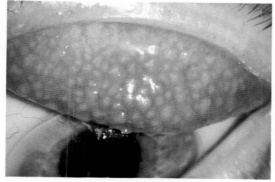

Figure 8.21 Soft lens wear with papillary conjunctivitis. Note mucus at lower margin of upper lid.

These are also acute inflammatory cells and hypertrophy of the mucous membrane. It is important to differentiate between papillae and follicles. Papillae are essentially vascular formations that have been invaded by inflammatory cells, whereas follicles are new formations of lymphoid tissue with accessory vascularization (Liebowitz, 1984).

GPC may be caused by:

1. the mechanical trauma of the lens on the conjunctiva.
2. allergenic proteins on the lens surface, and
3. possibly the lens material (Mackie and Wright, 1978).

Treatment Many contact lens wearers do not possess suitable spectacles, or are unwilling to stop wearing their contact lenses, so that any treatment may have to be compatible with continued contact lens wear.

1. Stop the use of any eye drops or lens care solutions which may have caused the allergy.
2. Replace the lenses with new ones, or clean the existing lenses thoroughly, to remove all antigen from the surface and inside of the lens.
3. Clean lenses with a preservative free surfactant every night prior to using preservative free lens care solutions.
4. Sodium cromoglycate drops (Opticrom 4% US, Opticrom 2% UK) can be used 3–4 times daily without the soft contact lenses (Meisler, Berzins

and Krachmer, 1982), or twice daily (before and after soft contact lens wear) with continued lens wear. As the drops are preserved with benzalkonium chloride, the manufacturers do not recommend their use when wearing soft contact lenses. In practice we have not found any corneal changes, when the drops have been used inadvertently when wearing the lenses for many months. The drops will not make the papillae regress to any marked degree, and they usually remain for many months, if not years, before they eventually do regress. However the drops should stop the symptoms of itching and redness, and markedly decrease the amount of mucus produced, so that it does not interfere with soft contact lens wear. A good regime is to use the drops until a bottle is finished, and then stop the drops for a few weeks, but restart another bottle if the symptoms recur. Taking stock at the end of each bottle will avoid the unnecessary use of the drops. Many patients have used them intermittently over a year or more to control the symptoms effectively. Should the condition worsen, steroids can be used in conjunction with sodium cromoglycate, for short periods of two or three weeks, without the lenses. For excessive secretion of mucus acetylcysteine 5 or 10% drops may help as a mucolytic. If the symptoms persist, soft lens wear will have to be stopped and the sodium cromoglycate drops used three or four times daily until the symp-

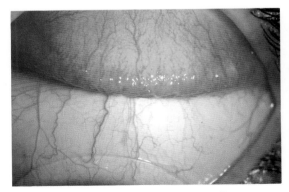

Figure 8.22 Soft lens wear with early papillary conjunctivitis in Zone 1. Note that in rigid lens wearers the papillae usually in Zone 3 first

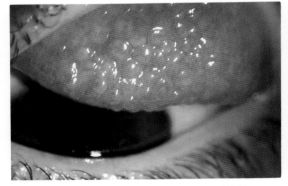

Figure 8.23 Giant papillary conjunctivitis (GPC)

toms abate. A period of several months is usually required before restarting soft lens wear. An alternative is to refit with RGP lenses.

Eventually, but usually only after several years, the papillae become smaller and whitish scars develop on the tops of the larger papillae (Figure 8.24). It is often difficult to know when to advise the patient to resume soft lens wear, but when the papillae are reducing, and discharge of mucus and tarsal inflammation have cleared, then lens wear may be restarted (Meisler, Berzins and Krachmer, 1982),

Contact lens superior limbic keratoconjunctivitis (CLSLK)

This syndrome which may occur in contact lens wearers, is a hypersensitivity reaction probably caused by thiomersal in care solutions and eye drops, used in conjunction with contact lenses (Wright, 1972; Wilson, McNatt and Reitschell, 1981; Miller, Brightbill and Slama, 1982; Wright and Mackie, 1982; Sendele *et al.*, 1983; Bloomfield, Jakobiec and Theodore, 1984, and Stenson, 1986).

Symptoms include a red, watery, and irritable eye occurring in a patient who has worn contact lenses for many months or years. Like GPC it occurs more frequently in soft lens wearers, and may cause photophobia with difficulty in keeping the eyes open.

Clinical findings Conjunctival hyperaemia and chemosis is confined to the area adjacent to the upper limbus, with marked limbal swelling which has a greyish colour and stains with fluorescein (Figure 8.25). Rarely a papillary response may occur under the upper lid from thiomersal, but is common in SLK of the Theodore type. Vascularization of the upper cornea is usually marked, with dilated vessels. An area of hazy epithelium in advance of the vascularization, has a tongue like process pointing towards the pupil, with a well defined margin where it adjoins the normal cornea (Figure 8.26). The best way of demonstrating thiomersal hypersensitivity is a challenge test of thiomersal containing drops in the eye, and noting the response. It is important that this is not done until the eye is quiet. Patch testing tends to be unreliable.

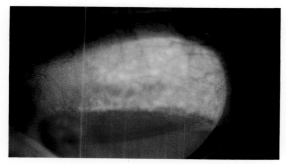

Figure 8.25 Limbal fluorescein staining with contact lens related SLK

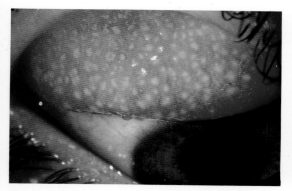

Figure 8.24 Resolving papillae with 'white heads' beginning to appear

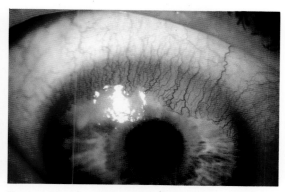

Figure 8.26 Contact lens related SLK from thiomersal

Treatment   Discontinue contact lens wear and in the early stages sodium cromoglycate 2% drops three or four times daily should resolve the condition (Confino and Brown, 1987).

When more advanced, topical steroids of varying potencies may also be required, but ensure that any eye drops used do not contain thiomersal. When the condition has cleared contact lens wear can be resumed, with new or thoroughly cleaned lenses, and thiomersal-free solutions and drops.

Corneal complications

Corneal oedema

This is not a common occurrence with soft contact lens wear, but can occur from corneal hypoxia. This is more likely to occur with low oxygen transmissibility thick soft contact lenses, when surface film reduces the transmissibility, and when the soft contact lens fit is tight. The hypoxia may lead to anaerobic metabolism, and an accumulation of lactates in the corneal stroma, to produce stromal oedema. Vertical striae in the posterior cornea are an early sign of stromal oedema (White and Miller, 1981). They are probably due to a buckling of the posterior stroma and Descemet's membrane, and increased swelling tendency of the posterior stroma (Polse, Sarver and Harris, 1975). Marked stromal oedema may

produce epithelial oedema detectable with the slit-lamp, and causing blurred vision with spectacles Any corneal epithelial defect may also lead to localized oedema. Polymegathism and reduced density of the endothelial cells predisposes to corneal oedema (Binder and Woodward, 1980).

Treatment   Lens wear should be discontinued until the oedema has cleared. The lens fit should be made flatter by reducing the TD or flattening the BOZR, and changing to a thinner lens with a greater oxygen transmissibility. Patients with endothelial changes require frequent checks for early signs of corneal oedema.

Corneal staining

Staining with fluorescein may be localized or generalized, and discrete or confluent punctate staining, and may occur from:

Mechanical trauma   This includes foreign bodies under a lens, and by film and/or deposit on the under surface of the lens (Figure 8.27). Corneal abrasions may be caused inadvertently by finger nails when inserting or removing lenses (Figure 8.28). Inadequate lid closure on blinking can lead to dessication of the lower part of the lens, which may produce punctate staining of the lower cornea. Peripheral arcuate staining is usually in the lower part of the cornea, from the edge of a small diameter lens, and particularly from the thicker edge of a high minus lens (Kline and De

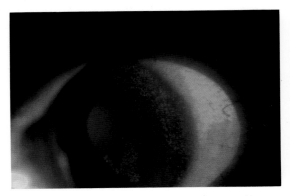

Figure 8.27   Corneal punctate staining from an FB under a soft lens

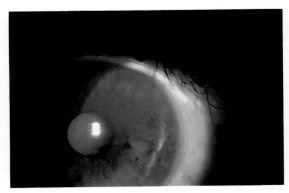

Figure 8.28   Corneal abrasion caused by a finger nail when removing a soft lens

Luca, 1981). A flat fitting lens can cause punctate staining of the central cornea. A damaged lens, or one of faulty manufacture, can cause punctate staining from the roughened area, or a defective edge, or bevel. A normal tear film will minimize these problems, but they will all be aggravated by a dry eye.

Hypoxia A tight fitting lens, or a lens which consistently leaves part of the cornea uncovered, can give rise to generalized or localized punctate staining and oedema respectively. Thick, lower water content lenses may lead to corneal hypoxia, with the oxygen transmissibility of the lens being further reduced by surface film and deposit.

Allergic and toxic reactions

Allergic reactions of the eye are usually associated with itching, excessive mucus production and conjunctival injection. One type of allergy is the hypersensitivity reaction which can occur from prolonged use of preservatives in contact lens solutions. Prolonged use of certain preservatives can also have a toxic effect on the cornea. Both conditions may produce coarse punctate epithelial staining, together with corneal epithelial opacities (Figure 8.29). It can be difficult to differentiate between toxic and allergic problems due to preservative induced complications. Thiomersal hypersensitivity will produce chronic irritation and redness soon after inserting lenses each day (Wilson *et al.*, 1981).

Treatment

Discontinue lens wear, and use preservative free rewetting eye drops. (See Chapter 4.) If more severe, steroid eye drops may be required, provided they do not contain thiomersal or chlorhexidine. When the condition has cleared, lens wear can be resumed, using lens care solutions without preservatives. Corneal pseudodendrites can occur from the use of thiomersal and chlorhexidine preserved solutions. They can mimic the dendrites of a herpes simplex keratitis (Margolies and Mannis, 1983; Udell *et al.*, 1985), but corneal sensation is usually normal. Pseudodendrites are usually bilateral, greyish slightly raised and intraepithelial infiltrates, which stain minimally. Resolution is generally slow after discontinuing contact lens wear, but the possibility of a herpes simplex infection must always be considered. From the same causes intraepithelial microcysts can be seen on the slit-lamp by retroillumination, which result from an extracellular oedema produced by rupture of the epithelial cell membranes, and occur mainly centrally. Discontinuing lens wear and the preserved solutions should resolve the problem. When the eye is quiet, a positive response to an ocular challenge of thiomersal or chlorhexidine is a useful way to diagnose the cause.

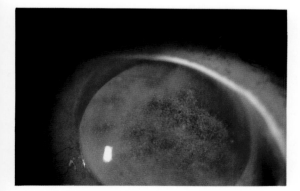

Figure 8.29 Toxic keratitis with punctate staining

Sterile corneal ulcers

These ulcers can occur anywhere in the cornea, and can resolve without any residual scar. They are thought to be secondary to an immune phenomenon (Rao and Saini, 1987). Appropriate investigations must be done to rule out any infective cause. Antibiotic therapy should be started prior to the investigation results being available. If no micro-organisms are found, topical steroids can be started gradually, usually with a good response. A sterile hypopyon can also occur, which should resolve in a few days, with mydriasis and cessation of lens wear.

Bacterial corneal ulcer

The causative bacteria can come from infected lenses, the lens case, the lens solutions, the hand of the wearer, or inadequate lens disinfection techniques (Figure 8.30). When a corneal ulcer is diagnosed corneal scrapings are done for culture and antibiotic sensitivity tests, before antibiotic therapy is started. The Gram-negative bacteria *Pseudomonas aeruginosa* is a common and damaging pathogen, which produces a mucopurulent discharge usually adherent to the corneal surface. A hypopyon is often an early occurrence, and rapid corneal melting with perforation can occur in only 1–2 days from the onset. Tobramycin eye drops for Gram-negative, and cefazolin eye drops for Gram-positive organisms, should be given, as intensive drops of both antibiotics (Laibson and Donnenfeld, 1986). Other organisms responsible for corneal ulcers are *Staphylococcus* spp., *Serratia marcescens*, and *Acanthamoeba*. The latter requires intensive propamidine, neomycin and polymyxin topical therapy, and may need keratoplasty to control a progressive infection. Early diagnosis and treatment are essential if serious complications are to be prevented (Cooper and Costable, 1977; Kracher and Purcell, 1978; Bohigian, 1979; Galentine *et al.*, 1984; Omerod and Smith, 1986; Chulupa *et al.*, 1987).

Corneal neovascularization

This is a common complication of soft contact lens and scleral lens wear, and less commonly from rigid lens wear. The new vessels originate from the marginal vessel arcades, and invade the superficial stroma. It is common for the vessels to invade up to 1–2 mm into the cornea, and no further (Figure 18.31), but unacceptable for the vessels to invade the cornea for more than 2 mm. Soft contact lens wear can cause corneal hypoxia, oedema, and keratitis, all of which may predispose to neovascularization (Ruben, 1981). It may also occur along the suture lines of a cataract operation, or keratoplasty, particularly when a soft lens is worn. A limited amount of neovascularization is acceptable, but a close watch must be kept on any vessels which seem to be advancing centrally and particularly following keratoplasty, when a vessel approaches the graft. Deep stromal vessels are uncommon, but may occur following corneal injury. They are more serious, as lipid

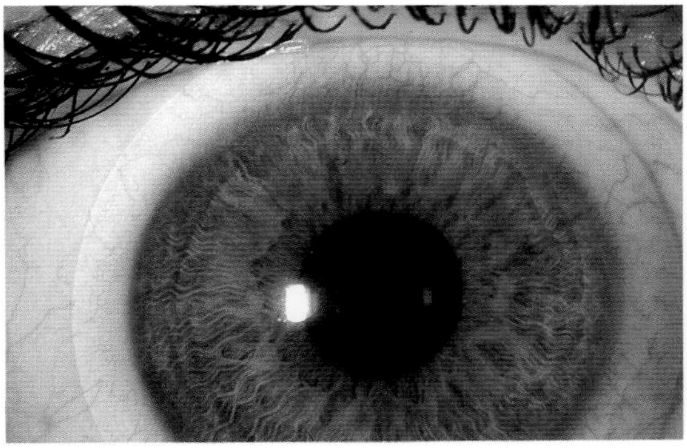

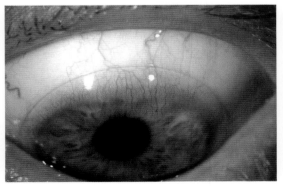

Figure 8.31   Acceptable amuount of corneal neovascularization

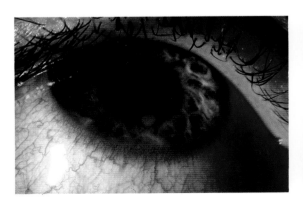

Figure 8.30   Corneal bacterial ulcer

Figure 8.32   Unacceptable amount of corneal neovascularization

infiltrates may occur, which can affect the vision, if central. The deep vessels may also cause corneal pannus, scarring, and intrastromal haemorrhages. Corneal neovascularization is one of the main reasons for reviewing soft lens wearers every six months, as the problem may be asymptomatic until it encroaches on the visual axis. If a soft contact lens wearer has neovascularization in excess of 1.5–2.0 mm, lens wear should be discontinued if possible (Figure 8.32). Often patients do not have any adequate spectacles, or are unwilling to stop lens wear.

Treatment

1. Fit a flatter lens, so long as it is stable on the eye.
2. Increase the lens water content.
3. Reduce the lens thickness, as much as possible.
4. Use weak (e.g. FML) topical steroids for short periods and under supervision.
5. When deep vascularization occurs, lens wear must be stopped.
6. When the vessels have emptied and regressed, lens wear can be restarted with close supervision.
7. Alternatively refit with an RGP lens.

Dry eye problems

These have been discussed in Chapter 2, but in a dry eye a soft lens will tend to dehydrate, and will be prone to develop surface film and deposit. Two factors are important in dealing with the problem.

Firstly, correct and adequate blinking – the importance of which cannot be overstressed. Many patients only 'flick blink', which leaves the lower half or more of the lens unwiped by the upper lid, and fails to clean or rehydrate the lens surface. Correct blinking entails complete lid closure without squeezing. The patient should be told to close the eyes, slowly and gently with the feeling that they are going to sleep, and then almost immediately open them again.

Secondly, lubricant eye drops – Adapettes (Chapter 4) contain thiomersal, and cannot be used for patients who have become allergic to this preservative. Unit dose unpreserved N-saline can be used but is expensive. Pilkington Barnes Hind produce Softmate rewetting drops which contain potassium sorbate as a preservative and are available in 15 ml and 60 ml bottles.

Iatrogenic problems

Inadvertent application of fluorescein or rose bengal stains when the patient is wearing a soft lens, causes immediate cosmetic problems. Neutral adrenaline (epinephrine) drops will cause yellow to brown discolouration over a period of time. Fluorescein and N-adrenaline can be removed with repeated hydrogen peroxide or intensive cleaning, but rose bengal staining usually means lens replacement (Figure 8.33).

References

ALLANSMITH, M.R., KORB, D.R., GREINER, J.V., et al. (1977) Giant papillary conjunctivitis in contact lens wearers. *American Journal of Ophthalmology*, **85**, 242–252

BERNSTEIN, H.N. (1973) Fungal growth into a Bionite hydrophic contact lens. *Annals of Ophthalmology*, **5**, 317–322

BINDER, P.S. and WOODWARD, C. (1980) Extended wear Hydrocurve and Sauflon contact lenses. *American Journal of Ophthalmology*, **90**, 309–316

BLOOMFIELD, S.E., JAKOBIEC, F.A. and THEODORE, F.S. (1984) Contact lens induced keratopathy. *Ophthalmology*, **91**, 290–294

BOHIGIAN, G.N. (1979) Management of infections associated with soft contact lenses. *Ophthalmology*, **86**, 1138–1141

CHULUPA, E., SWARBRICK, H., HOLDEN, B. and SJOSTRAND, S. (1987) Severe corneal infections associated with contact lens wear. *Ophthalmology*, **94**, 17–22

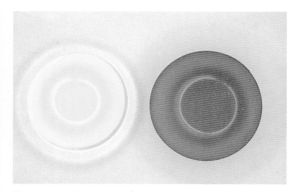

Figure 8.33 Iatrogenic soft lens contamination with fluorescein, and with rose bengal stains

CONFINO, J. and BROWN, S.E. (1987) Treatment of superior limbic kerato conjunctivitis with topical Cromolyn Sodium. *Annals of Ophthalmology*, **19**, 129–131

COOPER, R.L. and COSTABLE, I.J. (1977) Infective keratitis in soft contact lens wearers. *British Journal of Ophthalmology*, **61**, 250–254

DONSHIK, P.C., BALLOW, M., LUISTRO, A. and SAMARTINO, L. (1984) Treatment of contact lens induced giant papillary conjunctivitis. *The Contact Lens Association of Ophthalmologists Journal*, **10**, 346–349

GALENTINE, P.G., COHEN, E.J., LAIBSON, P.R., *et al.* (1984) Corneal ulcers associated with contact lens wear. *Archives of Ophthalmology*, **102**, 981–984

GREINER, J.V., FOWLER, S.A., and ALLANSMITH, M.R. (1984) Giant papillary conjunctivitis. In *The Contact Lens Association of Ophthalmologists Guide to basic science and clinical practice* (ed. O. Dabezies Jr), Grune and Stratton, New York, pp. 43.1–43.16

KLINE, L.N. and DE LUCA, T.J. (1981) Corneal staining. *International Ophthalmology Clinics*, **21**, 13–26

KRACHER, J.H. and PURCELL, J.J. (1978) Bacterial corneal ulcers in cosmetic soft contact lens wearers. *Archives of Opthalmology*, **16**, 57–61

LAIBSON, P.R. and DONNENFELD, E.D. (1986) Corneal ulcers related to contact lens use. In *Contact Lenses and External Disease* (ed. E.J. Cohen), *International Ophthalmology Clinics*, **26**, 3–14

LIEBOWITZ, H.M. (1984) Inflamation of the cornea. In *Corneal disorders, Clinical diagnosis and management.* (ed. H.M. Liebowitz), W.B. Saunders, Philadelphia, p. 271

MACKIE, I.A. and WRIGHT, P. (1978) Giant papillary conjunctivitis (secondary vernal) in association with contact lens wear. *Transactions of the Ophthalmological Societies of the United Kingdom*, **98**, 3–9

MARGOLIES, L.J. and MANNIS, M.J. (1983) Dendritic corneal lesions associated with soft contact lens wear. *Archives of Ophthalmology*, **101**, 1551–1553

MEISLER, D.M., ZARET, C.R. and STOCK, E.L. (1980) Trantas dots and limbal inflammation associated with soft contact lens wear. *American Journal Ophthalmology*, **89**, 66–69

MEISLER, D.M., BERZINS, U.J. and KRACHMER, J.H. (1982) Cromolyn treatment of giant papillary conjunctivitis. *Archives of Ophthalmology*, **100**, 1608–1610

MILLER, R.A., BRIGHTBILL, F.S. and SLAMA, S. (1982) Superior limbic kerato conjunctivitis in soft contact lens wearers. *Cornea*, **1**, 293–299

MONDINO, B.J., SALAMON, S.M. and ZAIDMAN, G. (1982) Allergic and toxic reactions in soft contact lens wearers. *Survey of Ophthalmology*, **26**, 337

ORMEROD, L.D. and SMITH, R.E. (1986) Contact lens associated microbial keratitis. *Archives of Ophthalmology*, **104**, 79–83

POLSE, K.A., SARVER, M.D. and HARRIS, M.G. (1975) Corneal oedema and vertical striae accompanying the wearing of hydrogel lenses. *American Journal of Physiological Optics*, **52**, 185–191

PRICE, M.J., MORGAN, J.F., WILLIS, W.E. and WASAN, S. (1982) Tarsal conjunctival appearance in contact lens wearers. *Contact and Intraocular Lens Medical Journal*, **8**, 16–22

RAO, G.N. and SAINI, J.S. (1987) Complications of contact lenses. In *Contact Lenses* (eds J.V. Aquavella and G.N. Rao), Lippincott, Philadelphia,' p. 217

RICHMOND, P.P. and ALLANSMITH, M.R. (1981) Giant papillary conjunctivitis. *International Ophthalmology Clinics*, **21**, 65–82

RUBEN, M. (1981) Corneal vascularization. *International Ophthalmology Clinics*, **21**, 27–38

SENDELE, D.D., KENYON, K.R., MOBILIA, E.F., *et al.* (1983) Superior limbic kerato conjunctivitis in contact lens wearers. *Ophthalmology*, **90**, 616–619

SPRING, T.F. (1974) Reaction to hydrophilic lenses. *Medical Journal of Australia*, **1**, 449–450

STENSON, S. (1986) Ocular surface disease complicating hydrophilic lens wear. *The CLAO Journal*, **12**, 158–164

TRIPATHI, R.C., TRIPATHI, B.J. and RUBEN, M. (1980) The pathology of soft contact lens spoilage. *Ophthalmology*, **87**, 365–380

UDELL, I.J., MANNIS, M.J., MEISTER, D.M., *et al.* (1985) Pseudodentrites in soft contact lens wearers. *The CLAO Journal*, **11**, 51–53

WHITE, P.F. and MILLER, D. (1981) Corneal oedema. *International Ophthalmology Clinics*, **21**, 3–12

WILSON, L.A., McNATT, J. and REITSCHELL, R. (1981) Delayed hypersensitivity to thimerosal in soft contact lens wearers. *Ophthalmology*, **88**, 804–809

WRIGHT, P. (1972) Superior limbic kerato conjunctivitis. *Transactions of the Ophthalmological Societies of the United Kingdom*, **92**, 555–560

WRIGHT, P. and MACKIE, I. (1982) Preservative related problems in soft contact lens wearers. *Transactions of the Ophthalmological Societies of the United Kingdom*, **102**, 3–6

YAMAGUCHI, I., HUBBARD, A., FUKUSHIMA, A., *et al.* (1984) Fungus growth on soft contact lenses with different water contents. *The CLAO Journal*, **10**, 166 –171

Further reading

COTTER, J. (1981) Soft contact lens testing on fresh water scuba divers. *Contact and Intraocular Lens Medical Journal*, **7**, 323–326

CUNHA, M.L., THOMASSEN, T.S., COHEN, E.J., GENVERT, G.I. *et al.* (1987) Complications associated with soft contact lens use. *The CLAO Journal*, **13**, 107–111

DURAN, J.A., REJOJO, M.F., GIPSON, K. and KENYON, K.R. (1987) *Pseudomonas* attachment to new hydrogel contact lenses. *Archives of Ophthalmology*, **106**, 106–109

EFFRON, N., BRENNAN, N.A., BENCE, A.S., *et al.* (1987) Dehydration of hydrogel lenses under normal wearing conditions. *The CLAO Journal*, **13**, 152–156

FOWLER, S.A. and ALLANSMITH, M.R. (1980) Evolution of soft contact lens coatings. *Archives of Ophthalmology,* **98**, 95–99

GREINER, J.V., KENYON, J.R. and KORB, D.R., *et al.* (1980) Mucus secretory vesicles in conjunctival epithelial cells of wearers of contact lenses. *Archives of Ophthalmology,* **98**, 1843–1846

GRUBER, E. (1979) Complications associated with spin cast soft contact lenses. *Ophthalmology,* **86**, 1129

HAMANO, H., KITANO, M.S., MITSUNGA, S., *et al.* (1985) Adverse effects of contact lens wear in a large Japanese population. *The CLAO Journal,* **11**, 141–147

JOHNSON, D.G. (1973) Kerato conjunctivitis associated with wearing hydrophilic contact lenses. *Canadian Journal of Ophthalmology,* **8**, 92–94

KORB, D.R., GREINER, J.V., ALLANSMITH, M.R., *et al.* (1983) Biomicroscopy of papillae associated with wearing of soft contact lenses. *British Journal of Ophthalmology,* **67**, 733–736

LIOTET, S., TRICLOT, M.P., PERDERISET, M., *et al.* (1985) The role of conjunctival mucus in contact lens fitting. *The CLAO Journal,* **11**, 149–154

MITRA, S. and LAMBERTS, D.W. (1981) Contrast sensitivity in soft contact lens wearers. *Contact and Intraocular Lens Medical Journal,* **7**, 315–322

9

Extended wear contact lenses

The term extended wear (EW) implies overnight wear. However, the terms continuous wear, permanent wear and prolonged wear have all had their advocates. It was realized in the early 1970s that soft lens materials were capable of allowing enough oxygen to pass through the lens to the cornea, from the upper palpebral blood vessels with the eye closed. Since these early soft lenses we now have RGP contact lenses which have even higher oxygen transmissibilities, and which are now also being used for EW. This chapter is mainly concerned with EW soft contact lenses, but RGP extended wear lenses will also be discussed at the end of the chapter.

The oxygen transmisibility of a soft lens depends on its water content and thickness (see Chapter 3).

Extended wear lenses can be used:

1. On a one or two weekly basis by patients who wish to wear contact lenses as an alternative to glasses, and do not wish to handle their lenses daily, or for whom this would be inconvenient. Wearing the lenses for longer without removal increases the incidence of complications.
2. On a two to three monthly basis by patients who need contact lenses for medical reasons, but have difficulty in handling them, e.g. aphakics.

Extended wear patient selection

This includes myopes and low hypermetropes, and excludes aphakics who are dealt with in Chapter 11. A patient who wishes to have cosmetic extended wear soft contact lenses will probably know about a successful wearer, who has extolled their virtues. They may also have read glowing reports about such lenses in the popular press. It is most important that they are told from the outset, that such lenses are not suitable for everyone. They should be informed of the possible complications which can occur, particularly if the lenses are used incorrectly. The greater cost of extended wear lenses, and the routine for follow up visits should be discussed. Patients should be advised to remove their lenses overnight for cleaning on a weekly basis, or at most every two weeks. It is quite likely though, that whatever they are told, they will wear their lenses for longer periods. Previously cosmetic patients were allowed to wear their EW lenses for two or three months, until an increase in the complications became apparent, but many patients only wish to have the convenience of wearing their lenses for a few days at a time. This group will tend to be younger than the aphakic group, and to have fewer problems. This is largely due to the higher incidence of dry eyes, and anterior segment infection in elderly aphakics. An aphakic soft contact lens will also have a greater central thickness, and a lower oxygen transmissibility.

The patient must have good motivation and hygiene, and be able to handle and look after the lenses satisfactorily. A myope or low hypermetrope who has previously been a successful daily wear soft contact lens wearer is usually a good candidate for extended wear. They should already be conversant with the handling and wearing of soft contact lenses, and their problems.

A patient's working conditions have a bearing on their suitability for wearing soft contact lenses,

particularly of the extended wear type. Occupations which involve the use of toxic sprays or fumes can be a problem, as they may be absorbed by the lenses, and cause a toxic keratitis. Working in an air conditioned room or home, and cooking can all produce problems with soft contact lenses.

Extended wear soft contact lenses to correct presbyopia are not yet available, and only a few toric extended wear soft contact lenses are available, which are in limited parameters, see Appendix 8 Table A8.5.

Ocular examination

Evidence of external infection should be looked for, such as blepharoconjunctivitis, meibomitis and dacryocystitis. The cornea should be examined for epithelial staining, stromal oedema, vascularization and infiltrates or opacities, and any pathology recorded. It is particularly important to evaluate the tear film, by examining the tear meniscus above the lower lid margin, first without and then with fluorescein. An inadequate tear meniscus, or a tear break up time of less than 10 seconds, is a possible contra-indication to EW soft contact lenses. In patients who have undergone plastic surgery to their lids, or a face lift, evidence must be sought for any corneal drying problem at night.

The patient must be able to blink normally, and to have complete lid closure with each blink. Patients with incomplete blinking are unsuitable for extended wear soft contact lenses, particularly if they have a wide interpalpebral fissure, which will cause excessive drying of the lens, as well as an increased risk of lens loss. In dry conditions a soft contact lens, particulary a thin low water content lens can lose a significant amount of water, so that the lens fit will tighten. It is also important to examine the conjunctivae of the upper lids for papillae. A few papillae are a common finding particularly in younger patients, and are not a contra-indication to extended wear lenses. Diminished corneal sensitivity is a possible problem for wearing extended wear lenses, and a marked decrease in corneal sensitivity is a definite contra-indication, as corneal sensitivity is essential for the early recognition of pain in the eye.

Extended wear soft contact lens selection

The choice lies between high, middle and low water content soft contact lenses. Table A8.4 in Appendix 8 shows the specifications of some of the lenses available. The high water content lenses (70–80%) are more suitable when there is doubt about possible tear film deficiency and where good oxygen transmissibility is required. Examples are the Permalens, Sauflon 70% and Sauflon PW 79%. Due to their fragility, high water content lenses are unsuitable for frequent lens removal, and have an increased susceptibility to produce surface film and deposits.

The middle water content lens (Hydrocurve II 55%) is much thinner, and is a tougher material suitable for frequent lens removal.

The low water content lenses (45% and below) are made much thinner in order to have sufficient oxygen transmissibility. They can be more difficult to handle, but are well tolerated, and more resistant to deposit formation. The low or middle water content lenses are satisfactory for most patients, as well as the Sauflon 70% lens. The other higher water content lenses are better for borderline dry eyes, and when maximum oxygen transmissibility is required. Being thicker they should also correct more corneal astigmatism. See Table A8.4 in Appendix 8.

The Toric Hydrocurve II 55% lens can be used for extended wear, provided the parameters available suit the astigmatic requirement. See Table A8.5 in Appendix 8.

Fitting cosmetic extended wear soft contact lenses

Having chosen the type of lens, manufacturers usually provide a guide to the initial choice of parameters. There are now some very thin lenses which are available in just one fit, i.e. one BOZR only, and several that are only available in flat or steep fits only. Further adjustments to the fit are made by varying the overall diameter of the lens. If no manufacturers' guide is available, the initial BOZR chosen should be about 0.50 mm flatter than the flattest K reading and as near as possible

to the estimated power required for a 13.00 mm TD lens, but up to 1 mm flatter for a 14.50 mm TD lens. If possible the lens should then be allowed to settle on the eye for half an hour, and the fit assessed. (See Chapter 8 for assessment of soft lens fit.)

An over refraction is done, and the lens changed for one of different power if necessary. A small amount of residual astigmatism which cannot be corrected with spherical power lenses, can possibly be corrected by changing to a lens with a greater central thickness. The alternative is a soft toric EW lens, provided the satisfactory parameters are available. (See Chapter 10 on toric lenses.)

Before taking away their lenses, patients must be taught how to insert and remove them, and how to look after them. (See Chapter 8.)

There are some patients who desperately wish to wear contact lenses but who are totally unable to insert them themselves. It is safe to wear lenses so long as the patient can remove them. They can arrange for a friend or relative to insert them when necessary, and provided the lenses have been cleaned and disinfected. The patient must be given full written instructions on the care and wearing of their lenses, including what to do in an emergency. They must be aware of the importance of the symptoms of blurred vision, redness, discharge and irritation, and that they must remove a lens and contact their ophthalmologist if any of these symptoms persist for more than a few hours. It should be stressed to the patient that they should never go to bed with a lens on a red eye, and that they should examine their eyes carefully every morning, for any signs of redness. Many patients do not like 'to worry their doctor', and hope that any problem will resolve tomorrow. This attitude must be eradicated for everyone's peace of mind.

Follow up visits

Initially patients should build up their wearing time and remove the lenses every night for the first week, when they should have their first checks visit. If there are no problems, they can wear their lenses overnight, but must remove them the next night for cleaning and disinfecting. They can then wear their lenses for two nights before overnight removal, and continue this progression until they are wearing their lenses for a week at a time. They should then have a regular night once a week when they remove, clean and disinfect their lenses and replace them the following morning.

The next checks should be at two to four weeks, two months, and then every three to four months. After one year of successful lens wear, the visits can be made at about six-monthly intervals.

These suggestions are dependent on there being no problems. Should problems arise, the patient must be seen as soon as possible. At all visits it should be emphasised to the patient that at the first sign of any redness, discomfort, blurred vision, or discharge in an eye, the lens must be removed immediately. If the symptoms do not clear up within a few hours, an ophthalmologist should be contacted.

At each visit the vision should be checked, in case the lens power needs to be changed. A lens which has surface film or deposits may make the patient artificially more myopic. Cleaning the lens, or a new lens to the same specifications, should restore the vision to normal again. If in doubt about the power of a lens, it should be thoroughly cleaned and then the vision retested with the clean lens on the eye.

The lens fit should be checked, and it is important to change the lens for a looser fit, if it seems to be too tight. The fit should be as loose as possible, provided the lens is comfortable and the vision good. It is always better to err on the side of a loose fit, to avoid the serious problems that can be caused by too tight a fit. The fit can be assessed with the slit-lamp, and the lens should centre well, and move about 1–2 mm with each blink. The edge of a tight lens can produce conjunctival indentation (Figure 8.7). Both lens surfaces are examined for surface film and deposits.

There can be some surface film and deposit on the under surface of the lens, which can abrade the cornea as the lens moves (Figure 8.16).

Patients should be given their next appointment before leaving the practice, and should be contacted if they do not keep it.

Care of the lenses has already been dealt with in Chapter 4.

Disposable extended wear soft lenses

Disposable EW soft lenses (Vistakon Acuvue) are becoming available in the USA and the UK at the time of writing.

This new approach has been well devised by the manufacturers. Patients wear a lens for a one or two-weekly period, and then discard the lens for a new one. There is a cost differential in favour of weekly wear lenses, which only costs 50% above that for a supply of two-weekly lenses. Basically, the complication rate should decrease the more frequent the lens change. The BOZR is 8.8 mm and the TD 14 mm only, so that they are 'one fit' lenses. Water content is 58%, and the CT for −3.00 DS is 0.07 mm.

Advantages of Acuvue disposable soft lenses

1. Elimination of all lens cleaning and disinfecting solutions.
2. Almost total absence of lens film and deposits.
3. Consistently clearer and sharper vision.
4. Less risk of conjunctival and corneal infection.
5. Lost lenses can be replaced immediately from patient's own stock.
6. Probable reduction in papillary conjunctivitis.
7. No preservative related solution problems. Care must still be taken with possible preservatives in rewetting drops.
8. The lenses are consistently accurate, as they are moulded in a constantly wet state. This eliminates the variations which can occur in lenses produced by hydrating the lens after lathe cutting in the dehydrated state.
9. Each lens is packed in a peel back soft plastic envelope in sterile normal saline, with a shelf life of four years. A plastic box contains six lenses. The patient is supplied with lenses on a three monthly basis, which they collect at their three monthly review with the clinician.

Disadvantages of Acuvue disposable lenses

1. The lenses are only available in powers from −0.5 to −6.0 DS, but this will be extended.

2. Due to their thinness, some patients may find them difficult to handle.
3. Also due to their thinness they will not correct corneal astigmatism, and any patient with more than 0.25 DC may not find their vision acceptable.
4. The lens fit may not be satisfactory for some patients.

Fitting schedule

After instruction on handling the lenses the patient has a 'starter pack' of six lenses for each eye. The patient is then seen again two weeks later for an initial check, and if all is well, after another four weeks, and a three months supply of lenses given to them. The patient is then seen at three-monthly intervals for a check, and to collect their next three months supply of lenses. After one year visits are made at six-monthly intervals or at any time should there be any problems.

Complications of extended wear soft contact lenses

These have been dealt with in Chapter 8 for daily wear lenses (see pages 67–77). In this chapter they will be listed, and any differences between daily wear and extended wear lenses discussed. The thinner higher water content lenses used for extended wear produce most of the differences, as well as the wearing of the lens overnight.

Tight lenses

See page 69.

Loose lenses

See page 70.

Damaged lenses

The higher water content lenses tend to be more fragile when handled. Lenses may be lost from the eye, and they may also become hidden under the upper lid. Some of the very thin lenses can be

difficult to find, particularly if they have rolled up. If a drop of local anaesthetic is instilled in the eye, and a fine glass rod swept under the upper lid, the lens should be found.

Blurred vision occurring on waking

This may be due to corneal oedema, or to surface film on the contact lens. Instilling N-saline drops in the eye, and gentle 'completely closed and open' blinking should resolve the problem, but may need to be repeated several times. The blurring can occur as an adaptive symptom, and stop after a week or two. If the lens becomes dehydrated on the eye during the night due to incomplete lid closure, it will become tight and uncomfortable. This should also be resolved with N-saline drops and blinking.

Dry eyes

This is a common problem, that may only be apparent when the patient is wearing extended wear lenses. The problem is more common in women, particularly at the menopause, and when on some contraceptive pills, decongestants and antihistamines. Incorrect, insufficient blinking will predispose to dry eyes, and this is likely to occur with prolonged periods of close work. More frequent correct blinking, with complete eye closure at each blink should help, together with the use of rewetting eye drops.

Surface film and deposits can occur on both surfaces of the lens, but are more common on the front surface. They are commonly protein or lipid, and occur mainly when there is a dry eye problem, with lack of the aqueous component of the tears. If a deposit is large a new lens will be needed, as it cannot be fully removed, and will leave a surface defect, which will rapidly attract more deposit.

Toxic keratopathy

Toxic keratopathy may occur, from absorption of toxic substances by the lenses, when being worn. Examples of this are smoke and aerosol sprays, which can produce a chronic condition, as the lenses are not being cleaned daily.

Conjunctival injection

This is a common transient symptom, usually due to dryness of the eyes, or to lens contamination. The lenses should be professionally cleaned and the cornea examined to exclude any pathology. The injection may be due to an allergy to preservatives in the contact lens solutions, or to an infectious cause.

Early corneal oedema

Early corneal oedema may only be detectable on the slit-lamp as folds in Descemets membrane. More advanced stromal oedema can be detected by an increase in corneal thickness. Epithelial oedema will cause some visual distortion with glasses, although the vision may not be so much affected with contact lenses. The cause may be hypoxic, and requires a lens with higher oxygen transmissibility.

'Tight lens syndrome'

This is the sudden onset of a red uncomfortable eye with some blurring of vision, usually in the early morning. It can occur at any time, and often with a lens which has previously been comfortable. The tendency of the pH of the tears to become more acidic during sleep, produces dehydration of the lens, which becomes tighter on the eye. The induced hypoxia produces anterior segment inflammation (McCarey and Wilson, 1982; Miranda and Garcia Castineiras, 1983). This can cause perilimbal oedema, progressing to epithelial oedema, iritis and raised intraocular pressure, if the lens is not removed immediately. Cycloplegics and steroids are required, and possibly treatment to reduce the intraocular pressure. Lens wear should be discontinued until the eye is quiet. If the lens had previously been satisfactory for some time, an identical new lens can be used. If however, there had been any previous incidents due to a possibly tight fit, a looser fitting lens should be substituted. The tight lens syndrome seems to be more common in aphakic than in myopic patients.

Hypersensitivity to preservatives

Hypersensitivity to preservatives in the contact lens solutions has been a problem in the past, but

should occur much less now with preservative free contact lens solutions. However, there are some patients still using solutions containing thiomersal, which can cause redness and irritation of the eyes. It is much less likely to occur with extended wear lenses, as the lenses are being cleaned less frequently (Figure 8.26).

Epithelial microcysts

These may occur in extended wear lens wearers, and seems to be a hypoxic change (Humphreys, Larke and Parrish, 1980). The contact lenses should be replaced by lenses with higher oxygen transmissibility, when the condition has fully cleared.

Papillary conjunctivitis

Papillary conjunctivitis under the upper lids may occur at any time, but is much less common in extended wear than in daily wear soft lens wearers (see Chapter 8 and Figure 8.22). Should it occur in extended wear patients lens wear may have to be discontinued, and 2% sodium cromoglycate eye drops used three or four times a day. More frequent lens removal and cleaning can be tried, but is rarely successful. The triad of itchy, red eyes, with excessive mucus discharge, should always suggest a papillary conjunctivitis.

Corneal neo-vascularization

This occurs commonly in extended wear soft lens wearers. It affects mainly the upper corneal periphery and is acceptable provided that the vessels do not extend more than 2 mm into the cornea, and that they remain superficial. Further encroachment requires the soft lens to be changed for one of higher oxygen transmissibility, and a change to daily wear if possible (Figure 8.32). Should the neo-vascularization not regress, soft lens wear should be discontinued, and a high RGP lens be tried.

Infective conjunctivitis

Infective conjunctivitis caused by bacteria, viruses, or fungi can occur at any time. A red eye particularly with a discharge, is the danger signal for the patient to remove the lens immediately, and see an ophthalmologist. Treatment consists of

appropriate investigations and thereapy. When the eyes are quiet again, it is best to restart contact lens wear with new lenses, and not rely on having the previously infected lenses cleaned and sterilized.

Corneal ulcers

Corneal ulcers occurring in extended wear soft contact lens wearers can be sterile or infected, but all corneal ulcers should be considered infected until proved otherwise (Adams *et al.*, 1983; Weissman *et al.*, 1984). Sterile ulcers are usually due to an immune response, and when investigations have ruled out any infection they may be treated with steroids. An infected corneal ulcer is an extremely serious complication of extended wear lenses. If the lens has not already been removed, it should be removed with sterile conditions and cultured. Corneal scrapings should be taken, and the appropriate bacteriological investigations done. Urgent treatment should be started immediately and changed if the investigation results suggest otherwise.

Most bacterial corneal ulcers which are not associated with contact lens wear are caused by staphylococcal organisms, whereas those associated with extended soft contact lens wear, are often caused by Gram-negative bacilli, especially *Pseudomonas* (Wilson, Schlitzer and Ahearn, 1981; Baum and Boruchoff, 1986).

Acanthamoebic keratitis can occur particularly when patients make up their own saline using distilled water. Corneal biopsy will confirm the diagnosis, and treatment consists of intensive topical neomycin, polymyxin, miconazole and propamidine isethionate (Moore *et al.*, 1985).

Silicone rubber lenses for extended wear

Silicone rubber lenses have been used in North America, but no so much in Europe. Because of their extremely high oxygen permeability they are suitable for extended wear. However, their disadvantages are:

1. They have a hydrophobic surface, and have to be surface treated to make them comfortable to wear.

2. The lens surface attracts deposits, particularly lipids, making them difficult to keep clean.
3. A lens adhesion problem may occur, when the lens will not move on blinking. The lens must then be removed with great care or the corneal epithelium may be removed with the lens. Before attempting to remove the lens, the eye should be irrigated copiously with N-saline drops.
4. They will not correct much astigmatism.

Silicone rubber lenses which are currently available are the Wohlk Silflex lenses from West Germany, and Danker Sila Rx lens in the USA. The lenses should be fitted slightly flatter than the flattest K reading, and should show 1–2 mm of movement on blinking. If the lens moves excessively and displaces from the cornea, a steeper fit is needed. However, one should aim for the flattest lens which will centre satisfactorily and which will give stable vision.

High *Dk* RGP lenses for extended wear

There are now several high *Dk* RGP lens materials available, which are suitable for extended wear (Table A8.1 in Appendix 8).

The reasons for using an extended wear RGP lens rather than a soft contact lens are:

1. For a dry eye problem and in dry environments.
2. If corneal infection is likely, or has occurred with a soft lens.
3. When infective keratoconjunctivitis has occurred.
4. When there has been frequent loss or breakage.
5. When rapid formation of surface film and deposits occurs with soft lenses.
6. When vision is variable and unreliable.
7. For corneal neo-vascularization.
8. For giant papillary conjunctivitis, as Opticrom drops can be used with RGP lenses.

The possible advantages of extended wear RGP lenses over soft lenses are:

1. Very high oxygen transmissibilities are possible.
2. There is a good tear pump action.

3. Less risk of infection.
4. Some visual improvement.
5. Fewer corneal problems.
6. Smaller overall diameter, which is useful when treating corneal neovascularization
7. No lens dehydration.
8. No lens absorption.
9. Usually fewer deposit problems.
10. Easier lens maintenance.
11. Longer lens life.
12. Less expensive

The possible disadvantages of extended wear hard lenses over soft lenses are:

1. Increased risk of lens loss.
2. More difficult to fit.
3. 3 and 9 o'clock staining.
4. Foreign body under lens problem.
5. Lens warpage.
6. Lens breakage, particularly with reduced front optic plus lenses.
7. Possibility of lens adhesion problem.
8. Increased lens awareness.

The Boston Equalens material may be taken as an example:

1. It has 2½ times the oxygen permeability of the Boston 4 material.
2. It has better resistance to mucus adhesion than PMMA.
3. There is a reduced tendency for deposit formation.
4. The dimensional stability is equal to Boston 2 and 4.
5. It has reasonable resistance to flexure, scratching and breakage.
6. It has effective ultraviolet light filtration.

In the use of extended wear rigid lenses, note the following:

1. Fit with a slight apical touch to minimize lens flexure. This helps to prevent the lens adhesion phenomenon, and improves vision particularly with an astigmatic cornea.
2. Fit a tricurve lens with an overall diameter about 9.50 mm and an axial edge lift of about 0.10 mm (Atkindon and Kerr, 1987).
3. Build up the wearing time gradually.
4. Frequent initial reviews.
5. For lens adhesion problems use copious N-saline drops

6. If overnight corneal oedema occurs, it should rapidly resolve with the eyes open, and with correct, adequate blinking.

High *Dk* RGP lenses may have a place as extended wear lenses, particularly for overcoming some of the more serious problems which may occur with soft lenses. However, one is left with two major problems which are difficult to overcome. Firstly there is the increased lens awareness of a rigid lens, and secondly the problem of foreign bodies under lenses. Both these problems can be diminished by reducing the axial edge lift (Atkinson and Kerr, 1987) but there is a limit to this, as it will reduce tear flow under the lens. In myopia, should lens flexure not be correcting the corneal astigmatism, the centre thickness of the lens can be increased by 0.20 to 0.40 mm.

The complications of high RGP lenses are as described for RGP lenses in Chapter 7.

In the future RGP lenses may be used for EW, but this has not happened yet.

References

ADAMS, C.P., COHEN, E.J., LAIBSON, P.R., et al. (1983) Corneal ulcers in patients with cosmetic extended wear contact lenses. *American Journal of Ophthalmology*, **96**, 705–709

ATKINSON, T.C.O., KERR, C. (1987) The Kelvin Equalens design. *The Optician*, Jan 2, 20–29

BAUM, J., BORUCHOFF, S.A. (1986) Extended wear contact lenses and Pseudomonas corneal ulcers. *American Journal of Ophthalmology*, **101**, 372–373

HUMPHREYS, J.A., LARKE, J.R., PARRISH, J.R. (1980) Micro epithelial cysts observed in extended contact lens wearing subjects. *British Journal of Ophthalmology*, **64**, 888–889

MCCAREY, B.E. and WILSON, L.A. (1982) pH, Osmolarity and temperature effects on the water content of hydrogel lenses. *Contact and Intraocular Lens Medical Journal*, **8**, 158–167

MIRANDA, M.N. and GARCIA CASTINEIRAS, S. (1983) Effects of pH and some common topical ophthalmic medications on the contact lens Permalens. *The CLAO Journal*, **9**, 43–48

MOORE, M.B., MCCULLEY, J.B., LUCKENBACH, M.B., et al. (1985) Acanthamoebic keratitis associated with soft contact lenses. *American Journal of Ophthalmology*, **100**, 396–403

WEISMAN, B.A., MONDINO, M.D., PETIT, T.H., et al. (1984) Corneal ulcers associated with extended wear soft contact lenses. *American Journal of Ophthalmology*, **97**, 476–481

WILSON, L.A., SCHLITZER, R.L. and AHEARN, D.G. (1981) Pseudomonas corneal ulcers associated with soft contact lens wear. *American Journal of Ophthalmology*, **92**, 546–554

Further reading

BINDER, P.S. (1979) Complications associated with extended wear soft contact lenses. *Ophthalmology*, **86**, 1093–1101

BINDER, P.S. (1983) Myopic extended wear with the Hydrocurve II soft contact lens. *Ophthalmology*, **90**, 623–626

BINDER, P.S. and WOODWARD, C. (1980) Extended wear Hydrocurve and Sauflon contact lenses. *American Journal of Ophthalmology*, **90**, 309–316

FELIUS, K. and VAN BIJSTERVELD, O.P. (1984) Effect of sodium cromoglycate on tear film break-up time. *Annals of Ophthalmology*, **16**, 80–82

FONN, D. and HOLDEN, B.A. (1986) Extended wear of hard gas permeable contact lenses can induce ptosis. *The CLAO Journal*, **12**, 93–94

LARNER, L. (1983) Extended wear contact lenses for myopes: a follow up study of 400 cases. *Ophthalmology*, **90**, 156–161

LEMP, M.A. and GOLD, J.B. (1986) The effects of extended wear hydrophilic contact lenses on the human corneal epithelium. *American Journal of Ophthalmology*, **101**, 274–277

MAGUEN, E., NESBURN, A., VERITY, S., ROSNER, I. (1984) Myopic extended wear contact lenses in 100 patients. A retrospective study. *The CLAO Journal*, **10**, 335–340

ROBIN, J.B., NOBE, J.R., SVAREZ, E. et al. (1986) Meibomian gland evaluation in patients with extended wear soft contact lens deposits. *The CLAO Journal*, **12**, 95–98

SMOLIN, G., OKUMOTO, M. and NOZIK, R.A. (1973) The microbial flora in extended wear soft contact lens wearers. *American Journal of Ophthalmology*, **88**, 543–547

START, W.J., MARTIN, N.F. (1981) Extended wear contact lenses for myopic correction. *Archives of Ophthalmology*, **99**, 1963–1966

10

Correction of astigmatism and presbyopia

Correction of astigmatism

It has been estimated that 25% of all prospective contact lens wearers have an astigmatism of 1.25 dioptres or more (Holden, 1975). A spherical PMMA lens can correct 4.0 dioptres of corneal astigmatism satisfactorily, and sometimes more. However, a spherical soft lens, or high GP rigid lens which can flex, may require one or both surfaces toric, to correct the vision adequately. True residual astigmatism is when the astigmatism found on refraction, is different from the corneal astigmatism found on keratometry. The cause is intraocular; the lens may be tilted, off axis, or toric in curvature; or the corneal back surface may be toric. If there is no astigmatic refractive error, but a toric corneal curvature as measured with the keratometer, the corneal astigmatism must be equal and opposite to an intraocular astigmatism, which it neutralizes. A spherical hard lens will neutralize the corneal astigmatism only, leaving a residual astigmatism. However, a soft lens, by moulding to the toric corneal curvature, will not produce any residual astigmatism. Toric lenses can be difficult to manufacture accurately and to fit successfully. The cost of each lens and the number of lens changes which may be required to obtain an acceptable result, make them expensive to use.

Toric lenses are used:

1. To improve the vision when a spherical lens is unsatisfactory.
2. To improve the stabilization of a lens on a toric cornea.

Toric PMMA corneal lenses

Spherical PMMA corneal lenses flex minimally on the eye, unless they are extremely thin, and can correct a large amount of corneal astigmatism provided a stable fit can be obtained. When the mean K reading is in the middle range, i.e. 7.5–8.0 mm try a spherical bi-curve PMMA lens with a BOZR just flatter than the mean K reading, BOZD about 7.0 mm, and a TD about 9.0 mm. For steeper corneas a smaller BOZD e.g. 6.0 mm, and a smaller TD e.g. 8.0 mm may produce a more stable fit. Thin high minus lenses may produce flexing and reduce vision. Should the lens edge abrade the cornea, the TD should be reduced, and/or the edge uplift increased. Corneal astigmatism up to 4.0 dioptres can usually be corrected satisfactorily with a spherical PMMA lens.

If the fit of the lens is unsatisfactory either a peripheral toric back curve, or a fully toric back curve may be required.

Peripheral toric back curve lenses

These may be used to correct the lateral slide (usually temporal), from 'astigmatism against the rule' (+ cylinder at 180°), which often occurs following a cataract operation with a usual superior 180° incision. The back optic zone is spherical, with an 8.0 mm BOZD, and a TD of 10.00 mm. The peripheral curves are made 1.0 and 0.5 mm flatter respectively than the BOZR.

e.g. C2 7.60 (8.00)/8.60 × 8.10 (10.00)

The larger BOZD and TD are more satisfactory with aphakic lenses. Ideally a toric periphery trial lens should be used to assess the fit. A smaller BOZD e.g. 7.0 mm, and smaller TD e.g. 9.0 mm may be required for myopic lenses.

Fully toric back curve lens

When corneal astigmatism is greater than 3 or 4 dioptres, a fully toric back curve lens may be needed to stabilize the lens. The two BOZRs should be made: 1. slightly steeper than the flattest K reading, and 2. slightly flatter than the steepest K reading with the usual amount of flattening (depending on the material used) for the toric peripheral curves.

   e.g. K readings 8.20 at 180/7.40 at 90.
   C2 toric 8.10 × 7.50 (7.00)/9.10 × 8.50 (9.00)

If there is insufficient venting under the lens, either a central 0.2 mm fenestration may be made, or if a new lens has to be ordered, the BOZRs can be flattened, and the BOZD made smaller e.g. 6.0–6.5 mm.

Trial lenses should be used to assess whether any residual astigmatism remains on over refraction. These lenses should have the steeper meridian marked by two peripheral engraved dots, and the patient's lenses should be similarly marked.

Bitoric lenses

A bitoric lens has both toric front and back surfaces, and is required when a fully back toric lens produces residual astigmatism. The trial lens together with a diagram to show the position of the dots when the lens has settled on the eye, and with the over-refraction results, is sent to the laboratory for the final lens to be made. The fully toric back curve lens should stabilize the lens on the eye, so that the front toric curve is held in the correct position.

Front toric lenses

The residual astigmatism as assessed on refraction over the spherical lens, is put on the front surface of the lens with a spherical back curve. The lens is stabilized by a prism ballast of about 1.5 prism dioptres to prevent rotation (Figure 10.1). It is rarely necessary to truncate a hard lens for stabilization, and it may make the lens uncomfortable; nor is it necessary to fit a prism ballast lens to the other eye. A convenient way of marking the lens is a dot at the 6 o'clock periphery. If the lens does not orientate with the prism exactly vertical, this must be taken into account when ordering the axis of the front cylinder axis, as is described for toric soft lenses.

The prescribed lens is checked on the patients eye to assess the vision. If this is unsatisfactory, the refraction and cylinder axis may be incorrect, the latter being assessed by any rotation of the lens on the eye. If the lens rotation is constant, a new lens may be ordered with the cylinder axis rotated on the lens, to bring it into correct position on the eye, together with any other change in refraction which has been found.

Summary of correction of astigmatism with PMMA lenses

1. Always correct corneal astigmatism with a spherical lens if possible.
2. If the fit is unstable try a spherical lens with a toric periphery.
3. If the fit is still unstable, or there is residual astigmatism, try a fully toric back curve lens.
4. If there is still residual astigmatism, a bitoric lens is required.
5. Residual intraocular astigmatism requires a prism ballast front toric lens.

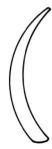

Figure 10.1   Toric soft lens prism ballast

Toric RGP lenses

RGP lenses can flex on the eye, particularly those with higher oxygen permeabilities. Because of their oxygen permeability they can be fitted tighter and larger than PMMA lenses, and this can give increased stability on an astigmatic cornea. Excessive flexure can be reduced by increasing the centre thickness of the lens. Toric curves may be required, as already discussed for PMMA lenses.

Toric soft lenses

Because of lens flexure a soft lens transfers practically all the corneal astigmatism through the lens to its front surface. The amount depends on the lens thickness, and increases with thinner lenses. Some patients will tolerate an uncorrected astigmatism if their vision is 6/9 or better. However, many discriminating patients, usually myopes, are often dissatisfied with even half a dioptre of uncorrected astigmatism. Less than 0.75 dioptre of astigmatism is best left uncorrected if possible, unless the patient requires the improved vision. The difficulty can be to ensure good stabilization of the lens, with minimal rotation on blinking and with eye movements. The toric surface may be on the front or the back of the lens, and it may be stabilized to prevent rotation by:

1. *Prism ballast* – usually about 1.0 to 1.5 prism dioptres (Figure 10.1), but the thicker lower margin of the lens can cause corneal hypoxia.

2. *Truncation* – which may be single or double, and used with or without prism ballast. The lens tends to settle on the eye with the lower truncation parallel to the lower lid margin (Figure 10.2). The lens may be unstable when truncation is used with oblique cylinders, due to the uneven lens thickness. Some patients are unduly sensitive to the lower edge of the lens bumping against the lower lid margin on blinking.

3. *'Thin Zone stabilization'* – by means of thinning the front surface of a large lens to reduce its thickness above and below (Grant, 1986). The thinner zones will lie under the upper and lower lids, resulting in a thinner and well tolerated lens (Figure 10.3). This is also known as a 'Slab Off' design in North America.

Small raised areas at the 3 and 9 o'clock lens peripheries, which align with the lid margins, have recently been introduced (Figure 10.4).

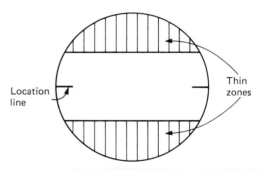

Figure 10.3   'Thin Zone' stabilization of a toric soft lens

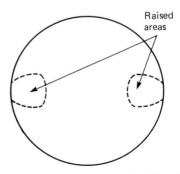

Figure 10.4   3 and 9 o'clock raised stabilization areas on a toric soft lens

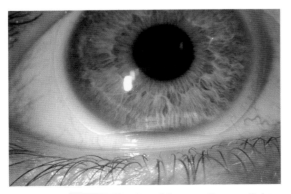

Figure 10.2   Truncated toric soft lens settling parallel to the lower lid margin

Best results are usually obtained with vertical or horizontal cylinders, and oblique cylinders can be difficult, if not impossible to stabilize (Maltzman and Rengel, 1985).

Most toric soft lens designs currently employed by manufacturers, use prism ballast with or without a single truncation, but double truncation alone is sometimes used. Toric soft lenses are either marked peripherally with single engraved lines at the 3 and 9 o'clock position, or else with one or more lines at 6 o'clock (Figure 10.5). For up to 4.0 dioptres of corneal astigmatism a large TD lens (15.0 mm) with upper and lower thin zones, and a toric front surface, are reliable e.g. Weicon T. For astigmatism above this amount a back toric lens should give a better result. The 'thinned zone' lenses are usually very comfortable (Table A8.5 in Appendix 8).

When fitting a front toric soft lens, it is important to establish the correct BOZR and TD, and trial lenses are essential for this. For the larger TD of 15.0 mm used for the 'Thin zone stabilization' lens, start with a BOZR 1.2 mm flatter than the mean K reading and assess the fit, as for a spherical soft lens. The lens is changed if necessary, and an over refraction is done. This is recorded in the minus cylinder form, together with the axis at which the engraved horizontal reference lines consistently align. Alignment within 20° of the horizontal or vertical is usually a good omen. Should the alignment not be at 180° or 90°, this must be allowed for when deciding the axis for the front toric curve. Several manufacturers provide a simple axis dial to aid this calculation (Figure 10.6). If the lens, when viewed on the eye, rotates in a clockwise direction, the degree of rotation is added to the cylinder axis in minus form, and subtracted if the lens rotates anticlockwise. When the patient is wearing the lens it may settle at a different alignment, and providing this is consistent, a new lens is ordered with the altered front toric axis. Toric soft lenses are prone to develop surface film and deposits, due to the absence of lens rotation, and may need more frequent cleaning, particularly with protein remover enzyme tablets.

Back surface toric soft lenses are made by some manufacturers, such as Hydrocurve II lenses which are only available in limited cylinder parameters. Others such as the Wohlk Hydroflex MT or TS can be made with cylinder powers from 0.5 to 6.0 dioptres. The parameters for the best fitting spherical lens are found, and the second radius of curvature for the toric back curve worked out from a table supplied by the manufacturer. The Hydroflex MT is stabilized by 1.5 dioptre prism ballast, and the Hydroflex TS lens has a 1.0 dioptre prism ballast, with an inferior truncation for stabilization (Gasson, 1980).

When a conjunctival draining bleb is present at 12 o'clock a superior upward curved truncation will aid stabilization, and prevent pressure on the bleb (Astin, 1987).

Hard/soft contact lenses

A recent addition to lenses for the correction of astigmatism is the Saturn II lens which has an 8 mm RGP centre, and a soft 25% water content peripheral flange. BOZRs are from 7.2 to 8.2 mm in 0.1 mm steps, the TD 14.3 mm, and the powers available from +6 DS to −13.0 DS in 0.25 DS steps.

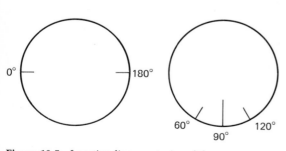

Figure 10.5 Location lines on toric soft lenses

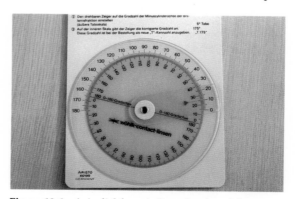

Figure 10.6 Axis dial for misaligned toric soft lenses

There were initial problems with the hard/soft junction but an improved version of the lens should soon become available.

Patient management

The various types of contact lenses available for the correction of astigmatism should be discussed with the patient, in case the first lenses are unsuitable. Patients should be warned that the fitting period can take up to two months or even longer, and that 10–15% of patients may still regard their lenses as unsatisfactory. The financial situation must be discussed with the patient, so that the clinician is reimbursed for the money has has paid out for lenses (Maltzman, 1983).

Correction of presbyopia

Myopes will become presbyopic at an earlier age when wearing contact lenses as they will have to accommodate more than when wearing spectacles. The opposite is true for a hypermetrope, particularly with fully corrected contact lenses.

When a patient who wears contact lenses becomes presbyopic, and requires additional plus power for near, there are several solutions:

1. The near vision can be corrected by wearing reading spectacles on top of the contact lenses, which will give the clearest reading vision of all the various methods. The spectacles may be in the form of half eyes, full size reading lenses, bifocals with plano or an intermediate correction at the top, or progressive addition lenses.
2. For presbyopes who only require a small reading addition, both distance contact lenses can be overplussed slightly, to enable the patient to see for distance and near. It will depend on whether the patient can accept a reduction in the distance vision, and on their distance vision requirements. If the patient is a driver, spectacles to improve the vision for distance could be worn on top of the contact lenses.
3. Single vision lenses, with the dominant eye corrected for distance, and the other for near, may be tried. To discover which is the dominant eye, ask the patient to point to a distance object with both eyes open. If they then close each eye in turn, the one with which the finger looks nearest to the object, is the dominant eye. Some patients do not like having 'different vision' in the two eyes, but a surprising number find it perfectly acceptable. As a trial the two different corrections can be put in the spectacle trial frame for the patient to try. However, if the patient drives, and the presbyopic correction is strong, it is a good idea to provide spectacles to go on top of the contact lenses for driving, to correct the near vision eye for distance vision. An alternative is to provide the patient with an extra distance contact lens, for the eye which is corrected for near.

If the patient does not want to wear spectacles at all, then bifocal contact lenses will have to be tried. These are difficult to manufacture, and can also be difficult to fit. The best bifocal contact lens wearer is usually a patient who is successfully wearing single vision contact lenses, but is now presbyopic. They need to be highly motivated, and should have a definite requirement for both a distance and a near correction. They should preferably have a minimal amount of astigmatism, to obtain good vision. It is also helpful if they have worn bifocal spectacles satisfactorily. The prospects for bifocal contact lenses, would not be so good, if the patient has previously had problems with single vision contact lenses, or bifocal spectacles. The basic principles of bifocal contact lenses are the same for both hard and soft lenses, and they can be designed to give either simultaneous or alternating vision.

Simultaneous vision

With the simultaneous vision design, both distance and near parts of the lens have to be within the pupil area at the same time. The lens has to be fitted to centre well, and with minimal movement. The patient will see both distance and near at the same time. Depending on whether they are looking at a distant or near object, the brain will select the clear image, and ignore the blurred one. However, not all patients can manage to ignore the out of focus image, and cannot manage with this type of lens. The lens may be either:

1. *A concentric or annular bifocal* in which the central part of the lens is usually the distance correction, and the surround is the near vision correction (Figure 10.7). The Alges soft bifocal lens has the near addition in the centre, and is surrounded by a distance zone.
2. *An aspheric or progressive addition bifocal* where the plus power increases gradually from the centre to the periphery. The strongest near addition which is possible for this type of lens is about +1.5 DS. The aspheric lens seems to give better vision for distance, while the concentric lens tends to be better for near vision.
3. *A separate central diffractive zone* on the back of the lens, which gives two different focal powers with no specific near or distance zones or segments (Freeman and Stone, 1987).

Alternating vision

An alternating vision type of lens is designed so that on looking straight ahead, the distance correction is in front of the pupil. On looking down at close work the lower lid should push the lens up on the eye, so that the near correction is in front of the pupil. For the lens to move it must be fitted loosely, and the lower lid must be high enough, and not be too loose. The lens may be of two basic designs:

1. *A concentric or annular design* as already described, which usually has the distance correction in the centre, and must be fitted loosely so that it can move up on looking down.
2. *Segment bifocals* are similar to spectacle bifocals, in that the distance correction is above and the near correction below (Figure 10.8). As the lens must not rotate, prism ballast and possibly truncation must be used, similar to that used for toric lenses. The reading segment may have a crescentic or straight upper margin (Figure 10.9) ground on to the front surface and be made in one piece. The near vision addition, can alternatively be made of a fused segment of a higher refractive index material, on the back surface (Figure 10.10). The higher the reading

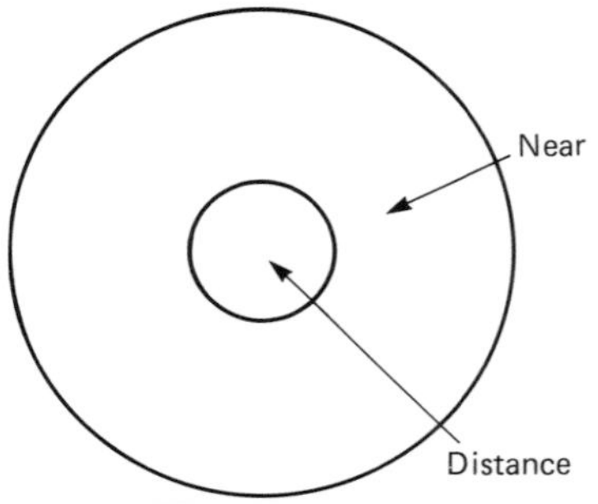

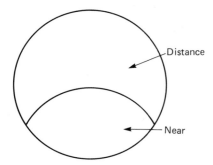

Figure 10.7   Concentric or annular bifocal lens

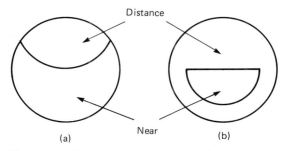

(a)   (b)

Figure 10.9   Reading segment shapes (a) crescentic (b) straight

Figure 10.8   Segment bifocal lens

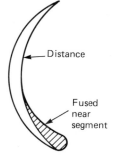

Figure 10.10   Fused bifocal segment of higher refractive index material

segment the better, so long as it does not interfere with the distance vision.

An alternating vision lens should give the best vision provided that:

1. The pupil is smaller than 4.0 mm in diameter in average indoor lighting conditions.
2. The lower lid margin is at the limbus or higher, and in good apposition to the globe.
3. The lower lid margin moves the lens upwards satisfactorily on looking down for near.

If these criteria are not fulfilled, a simultaneous vision lens can be tried, but the patient will probably tend to have some blurring of vision.

Bifocal rigid contact lenses

A *concentric rigid bifocal lens* can be tried as an *alternating vision* lens, but is less likely to move up on the eye when the patient is looking down. Increasing the lens overall diameter, and a truncation, may assist the lens movement. The lens needs to be about 9.0 to 9.5 mm overall diameter, and to have an alignment fit. Refraction for distance and near is done over the lens, and a lens ordered. The central distance zone diameter should be slightly larger than the average pupil size. Initially this would be made 4.0 mm for myopes, and slightly smaller for hypermetropes. Too small a central distance zone will give poor distance vision, and if this is so, the distance zone can be increased. The parameters which can be altered are the diameter of the central distance zone, the lens fit, the lens edge thickness (if too excessive) and the truncation.

A *concentric bifocal* can also be fitted as a *simultaneous vision* lens by fitting the lens more tightly, so that the distance part stays in front of the pupil. The central distance zone must be smaller than the pupil. This type of lens is not often used because of the poor quality of vision obtained, but it can also be made in an aspheric form, to give a progressive reading addition.

The recent Pilkington *Diffrax lens* is a simultaneous vision bifocal lens with a central back surface 5 mm diffractive zone, which can produce up to 3.00 DS reading addition. The lens must be fitted with some apical clearance to avoid contact of the central diffraction zone with the cornea (Freeman and Stone, 1987). Some adaptation is usually necessary to obtain the best visual result. There is often a lack of contrast for near, with a dark shadow behind printed words, and above or below a printed line. Print may also appear to stand out from the page, and flare may be experienced with night driving. All these effects should usually disappear within a few weeks, but some patients may continue to have problems. These lenses are easy to fit, and the use of trial lenses should give some idea of whether they are likely to be successful.

The *segment bifocal* usually gives improved vision, so long as it can be made to function properly. The design is similar to a spectacle bifocal lens, where the reading segment is below the distance area. Prism ballast and truncation help to keep the lens in the correct position, and assist the lower lid margin to elevate the lens on looking down. The lens is made from one piece of material, which has usually been PMMA, but gas permeable materials are being used more frequently. The lower reading curve may either be downswept or upswept, the latter giving better near vision should the lens rotate slightly.

The *fused segment* alternating vision bifocal lens has the reading segment made from a material of different refractive index, commonly styrene. The fused segment may have a straight upper margin, or be upswept, and the lens stabilized by prism ballast and truncation. The reading segment is often treated with a material which fluoresces with ultraviolet light, which enables the position of the reading segment relative to the pupil to be determined more accurately.

To fit rigid alternating vision segment bifocals it is important to have a fitting set of lenses of the same design as the lens to be ordered. The lens should be fitted loose enough to give adequate movement of the lens on looking downwards. When the lens has settled the position of the upper margin of the reading segment relative to the pupil lower margin is assessed. Ideally this should be just above the lower pupil margin for hypermetropes, and at, or just below, in myopes. The position will also vary according to the size of the pupil, and will need to be higher for larger pupils. According to how the lens settles on the eye, it may be raised or lowered by reducing the vertical diameter from the top, or from the lower truncated margin.

Bifocal soft contact lenses

Simultaneous vision may be obtained with a *concentric soft bifocal* which can have an aspheric back curve to give a progressive addition of near power towards the periphery. As the maximum effective reading addition is only about +1.5 DS, they are only suitable for early presbyopia. An example of such a lens is the Bausch and Lomb PA1. The Ciba Vision 38E Bi-Soft has a choice of two distance diameters, as well as two overall diameters, and a separate reading addition up to +3.00 DS. All these lenses should centre well on the eye, with minimal movement. This is easier to attain than in the case of hard lenses. The central distance zone diameter must be smaller than the pupil diameter. The Alges concentric bifocal lens is designed so that the central zone is for near vision, and can be either 2.12, 2.35 or 2.55, 3.0 and 3.5 mm in diameter. It is surrounded by a distance zone 8.50 mm in diameter. The reading addition powers are +2.00, +2.50, +3.00 and +3.50 DS (Gross, 1985). The near vision zone diameter should be increased if there are problems with close work. The reading addition needs to be +0.50 to +1.00 DS, greater than that required for spectacles. It is possible to have different near vision zone diameters on the two eyes, so that one eye may be better for distance, and the other for near.

Alternating vision may be obtained with a *crescent bifocal soft lens*, like that produced by Bausch and Lomb. This is lathe cut and has 45% water content with prism ballast and a notched truncation below.

There are two BOZRs, two TDs, reading additions of +1.50, +2.00 and +2.50 DS, and distance powers of −5.0 to +5.0 DS in 0.25 mm steps, and −5.5, −6.0, +5.5, and +6.0 DS.

To fit the lens, use the flattest BOZR and the estimated distance and reading corrections. The lens should centre well and the notch locate at 6 o'clock, with up to 15° rotation acceptable. The lens should move freely on the eye, and the top of the reading segment position near the lower margin of the pupil, when looking straight ahead. An over-refraction for distance and near is done, and the lenses ordered from these findings. Another similar lens is the Wesley–Jessen Durasoft 2 bifocal lens, which is also stabilized with prism ballast and truncation. It is available in one TD and BOZR, in two segment heights and in reading additions up to +2.75 DS.

Several factors determine the success rate for bifocal contact lenses. It is essential for the patient to have good motivation, and it helps if they have previously worn contact lenses. Younger presbyopic patients are usually easier to fit successfully, and there should be sufficient refractive error to need a distance and near correction. Patients who have long periods of close work, or who spend many hours looking at VDU screens may find bifocal lenses unsatisfactory. Important factors in bifocal wear are the pupil size, and the position and tension of the eyelids. With an alternating vision bifocal lens, a low positioning lower eyelid may not be able to push the lens up sufficiently on the eye on looking down for near. A loose lower eyelid will allow the lens to move down behind the lid on looking down.

A patient may require better vision for either near or distance, which cannot be satisfied by having a pair of bifocal lenses. A possible solution is for one eye to be corrected by a bifocal lens, and the other eye with a single vision near or distance lens. This can work well, particularly if a toric lens is needed on one eye only.

Better vision can be obtained with an alternating vision lens rather than a simultaneous vision type, providing the former will function satisfactorily. Soft lenses are more comfortable than rigid lenses, and have larger near and distance vision areas because of their larger overall diameters. Rigid bifocal lenses are not so much used now, but with the use of RGP materials for manufacture they may come back into favour again. None of the existing bifocal designs are successful in all patients, but most will be successful for some patients. The problem is to find out which design might be best for the individual patient.

References

Astigmatism

ASTIN, C. (1987) Three cases of fitting a superiorly truncated hydrophilic lens. *The Journal of the British Contact Lens Association*, **10**, 27–28

GASSON, A. (1980) A comparative appraisal of front and back surface toric soft lenses. *The Journal of the British Contact Lens Association*, **31**, 131–136

GRANT, R. (1986) Mechanics of toric soft lens stabilisation. *Transactions of the British Contact Lens Association* pp. 44–47

HOLDEN, B.A. (1975) The principles and practice of correcting astigmatism with soft contact lenses. *Australian Journal of Optometry*, **58**, 279–299

MALTZMAN, B.A. (1983) Management of astigmatism with toric contact lenses. *International Ophthalmology Clinics*, **23**, 33–56

MALTZMAN, B.A. and RENGEL, A. (1985) Soft toric lenses—an update. *The CLAO Journal*, **11**, 335–338

Presbyopia

FREEMAN, M.H. and STONE, J. (1987) A new diffractive bifocal contact lens. *Transactions of the British Contact Lens Association: Annual Clinical Conference*, **4**, 15–22

GROSS, M. (1985) A clinical evaluation of the Alges (Lefilcon A) Bifocal Contact Lens. *Canadian Journal of Optometry*, **47**, 174–176

Further reading

ANDRASKO, G. (1984) Bifocal Soft Lenses—A comparison. *Contact Lens Forum*, **9**, 53–56

ERICKSON, P. and ROBBOY, M. (1985) Performance characteristics of a hydrophilic concentric bifocal contact lens. *American Journal of Optometry, and Physiological Optics*, **62**, 702–708

MOLINAR, J. and CAPLAN, L. (1986) Clinical evaluation of two soft lens bifocals. *Journal of the American Optometric Association*, **57**, 684–686

MORRISON, R. (1986) Simultaneous Imagery Soft Bifocal contact lenses. *Transactions of the British Contact Lens Association Annual Clinical Conference 1986*, 76–80

11

Lenses for aphakia, infants and children

Aphakia

Most ophthalmologists now agree that an intraocular lens is the most satisfactory method of visual correction for aphakia, but a contact lens is preferable to spectacles when an implant is contraindicated. For unilateral aphakia uncorrected by an implant, a contact lens is the only way to obtain binocularity. In bilateral aphakia, many patients cannot use spectacles, due to the magnification induced, the smaller visual field, the peripheral field distortion, and the thickness and weight of the lenses. However, newer spectacle lenses which partially overcome some of these problems are now becoming available.

For those aphakics, without an implant, a contact lens will give the best vision. Correction may be by a daily wear PMMA, RGP or soft lens, or by an extended wear RGP or soft lens. For patients who cannot handle contact lenses, an extended wear lens will be required.

Extended wear soft contact lenses have been used to correct aphakia in the UK for over 15 years, and the problems which may occur are well known. Aphakic patients with EW soft contact lenses who have recurrent attacks of keratitis and corneal ulcers, should have their lenses discontinued. For bilateral aphakics who are relatively immobile, the improved aphakic spectacle lenses should be prescribed, and if they are active, secondary intraocular implants considered. For a unilateral aphakic the choice lies between an implant, or spectacle correction of one eye only, if a contact lens has to be discontinued. If a patient can handle a contact lens, then the lens of choice is a PMMA or low RGP lens. These lenses are well tolerated, mainly due to the reduced corneal

sensation of the upper half of the cornea, and by the fact that many aphakic patients have loose upper lids. Handling contact lenses may be a problem for bilateral aphakics, but provided one contact lens is fitted satisfactorily before the second cataract operation, most patients will manage well. If they rely on looking into a mirror to put a lens on the eye, then a pair of near vision spectacles, with the lens and lower part of the frame removed from one side, can be helpful (Figure 11.1).

It is important to remember when ordering aphakic contact lenses, to order the reading spectacles to wear with them also, so that when the patient comes for handling instruction, their spectacles are ready and they can see to read with their new contact lens. A +2.5 DS addition is the usual power required, as a +3.0 addition generally focuses too close.

PMMA corneal lenses

The most satisfactory form is usually a tri-curve lenticular design, with a peripheral minus carrier, and a total diameter of about 9.5 mm. The lenticular design will give a reduced central thickness of the lens, and thus reduce its weight. The minus carrier will aid attachment to the upper lid. However, the smaller front optic may produce flare from a large pupil, and particularly a keyhole pupil. Traumatic aphakia can often produce problems related to central corneal scarring and a distorted large pupil (Figure 11.2). For these patients a 'single cut' lens can be tried in which the front curve is continuous across the front surface.

A single cut lens may be better for small steep corneas, and narrow palpebral fissures, but if the lens drops excessively a minus lenticular lens should be used. A PMMA lens should correct all the corneal astigmatism. In practice a lenticular lens is almost always used.

Fitting of PMMA lenses

This can be undertaken as soon as the eye is quiet after operation, and all loose sutures removed. Use lenticular trial lenses the same total diameter as the final lens, and as near as possible to the final power. The initial lens should have a BOZR slightly flatter than the mean K reading. The fit is assessed for centration, lid adherence and movement, and the lens ordered in the usual way, as a tri-curve, with a BOZD of 7.5 mm or slightly larger depending on the size of the pupil. Lenticular lenses are usually ordered as 9.5 mm or more total diameter, to increase the lens stability, and to allow a large enough front optic. If 4.0 or more dioptres are in the trial frame on over refraction, the back vertex distance from the lens must be measured, and this allowed for in the final prescription from the Table in Appendix 4.

Note that the lens may be ordered as back or front vertex power from the manufacturer, but their computers normally work, on front vertex power. The junction thickness of a minus lenticu-

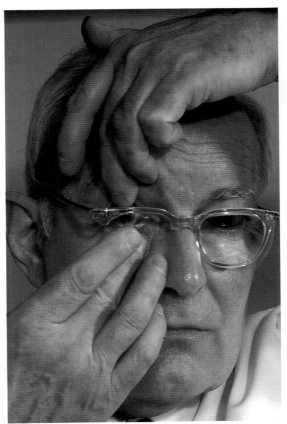

Figure 11.1   Bilateral aphakic patient using near vision spectacles with the frame removed on one side to aid placement of the first lens

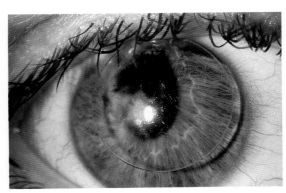

Figure 11.2   Traumatic aphakia with central corneal scarring and iridectomy

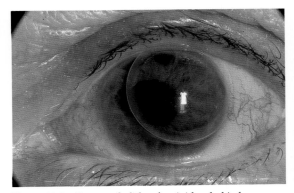

Figure 11.3   Temporal slide of a rigid aphakic lens

lar lens should be about 0.13 mm, as it will tend to break easily at the junction, if any thinner. If thicker, it will produce an increase in the centre thickness of the lens. The lens should be made from tinted material to assist location of the lens on the eye, or when dropped. A useful tint is a light grey, but a darker tint may be used if preferred by the patient.

When there is an astigmatism against the rule (plus cylinder at 180°) the lens may slide temporally on the cornea (Figure 11.3). This can usually be overcome by using a larger lens, with a larger BOZD and a toric periphery e.g.:

7.6 (8.0)/ 8.6 × 8.1(10.0)

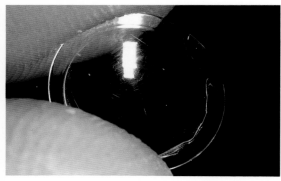

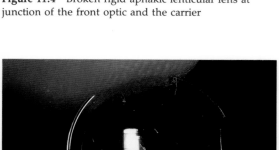

Figure 11.4 Broken rigid aphakic lenticular lens at junction of the front optic and the carrier

where the two peripheral toric radii are 1.0 and 0.5 mm flatter than the BOZR respectively.

A single cut lens may be preferable when a large or keyhole pupil produces ghosting or flare with a lenticular lens, or the lenticular lens may be made larger. The single cut lens can be smaller, i.e. 8.5 or 9.0 mm total diameter, and the edge can be thinner than for a lenticular lens, which may make it more comfortable to wear. A single cut lens which has a tendency to drop may produce corneal oedema with neovascularization below, and corneal warping. A single cut lens can be more difficult to remove from the eye. The lens may also tend to break or chip at the edge, while a lenticular lens will tend to break at the junction of the front optic and the carrier (Figures 11.4 and 11.5). Small chips and breaks are often not noticed by the aphakic patient until they have become quite large. Great care must be taken when fitting patients with draining blebs or iris prolapses, as trauma to the overlying conjunctiva could produce intraocular infection. The lens must avoid contact with such blebs or prolapses (Figure 11.6).

Rigid gas-permeable corneal lenses

RGP lenses may be required to prevent corneal oedema e.g., from endothelial dysfunction, or when a larger or tighter lens is required to obtain better stability. Silicone acrylate lenses e.g., Boston II or Polycon II, may be used, preferably of lenticular design, and need to be handled carefully

Figure 11.5 Piece missing from the edge of a rigid aphakic lens

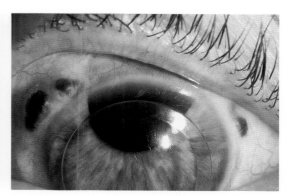

Figure 11.6 Iris prolapses in an aphakic patient wearing a rigid lens

as they are more prone to breakage, or scratching. The recent very high *Dk* RGP lenses are suitable for extended wear. It is important not to fit them too tight, and they should be fitted slightly flatter than the flattest keratometer reading, with minimal apical touch when checked with fluorescein. As extended wear hard lenses cannot usually be worn for as long as extended wear soft lenses without removal, they are only suitable for those patients who can handle them satisfactorily. They normally need to be removed for cleaning every one or two weeks.

Daily wear aphakic soft lenses

These are soft lenses with a water content from 38 to 50%, but the vision is not usually as good as with hard lenses, even with any astigmatism corrected by additional spectacles. They are suitable for patients who are able to handle them, and when stability is a problem with a rigid lens. Younger patients tend to prefer them, particularly when they lead an active life. Residual astigmatism may need to be corrected with glasses, and as the patient needs a reading correction, bifocals can be used.

Fitting of daily wear soft lenses

Use a trial lens with a total diameter of 13.50 mm and a BOZR depending on the keratometry, and determined from the manufacturers' table (see Table A8.2 in Appendix 8). The power should be as close as possible to the expected power required. After 15 minutes or so, when the lens has settled on the eye, it should move about 1–2 mm with each blink. The BOZRs of the lower water content lenses, e.g. pHEMA, are in 0.20 mm steps, while the higher water content lenses are usually in 0.30 mm steps. It is most important that the lens should not be fitted too tight. It is better to fit on the flat side, if the best fit is in between what the manufacturer supplies.

Problems of daily wear soft lenses

1. Lens surface film and deposits, including fungus growth
2. Damage by fingernails and by trapping the lens in the case

3. Loss when handling
4. Corneal neovascularization
5. Toxic keratitis
6. Bacterial conjunctivitis
7. Corneal ulcer

These are dealt with in Chapter 8.

Extended wear soft lenses

As many aphakic patients are not able to handle their lenses, an extended wear soft lens may be required. These lenses have a water content, from 55% up to 79%. Lenses should preferably be 70% water content and above, as they can be thicker, and will thus correct more corneal astigmatism. The lower water content lenses have to be made thinner to have an adequate oxygen transmission. The aphakic cornea seems to have a reduced oxygen requirement, and tolerates extended wear lenses very well.

Contra-indications to extended wear soft lenses for aphakia

1. Chronic infection such as blepharoconjunctivitis and dacryocystitis
2. Excessively dry eyes
3. Incomplete lid closure e.g. from facial nerve palsy and thyroid disease
4. Diminished corneal sensation
5. Poor motivation, compliance and hygiene
6. Inability to have a lens removed, or to see an ophthalmologist promptly when problems occur

Soft lenses which are suitable for extended wear in aphakia are listed in Table A8.4 in Appendix 8.

Extended wear lenses are available in different water contents, BOZRs and TDs. Start with a lens with an TD of 14.0–14.5 mm and BOZR of 8.3–8.5 mm and the estimated power on the eye. When the lens has settled for about half an hour, the fit is assessed. Ideally it should centre on the cornea with a 1–2 mm overlap all the way round, and should move 1.5–2 mm on blinking. Should the lens not move much, or at all, it should be changed for a flatter lens, and assessed again. Should the lens move excessively, particularly on looking upwards it should be changed for a

steeper lens. It is important that the flattest lens which will centre correctly should be chosen. If a lens is slightly too tight, it will become even tighter by the evenings when the eyes tend to be at their most dry, and the lens dehydrates and becomes tight on the eye. Allowance must always be made for this. An over refraction is done, and the lens changed for one of a different power if necessary. Full written instructions must be given to the patient, and they are provided with N-saline drops for rewetting the lens in the morning on awakening, and at any time during the day when necessary. It should be stressed to the patient that they must be seen immediately by an ophthalmologist, should they have a red or painful eye, and any blurring of vision or discharge, and it should be recorded in their notes that this has been done. A relative or friend should be shown how to remove the lens if it is necessary, and the procedure should be detailed in the written notes.

The patient should be seen the following day, when the lens should have fully settled on the eye. The fit is assessed with the slit-lamp and an over refraction is repeated, the lens power being changed if necessary. Any residual astigmatism can be put in spectacles, together with the spectacle reading correction. This can most conveniently be given as a bifocal lens, which the patient has probably been wearing previously. The next review should be at two weeks, one month, and then every three months, or at any time should there be problems. A common problem is the occurrence of film and deposits on the lens, and if this occurs in under three months, it is a good idea to see the patient every two months or so. If a lens becomes contaminated it will require changing, and a spare lens must always be kept in stock for the patient. Whenever a patient goes abroad, they should take a spare lens away with them, in case of problems.

Complications are the same as for other extended wear soft lens patients and have been dealt with in Chapter 9. However, aphakic patients are more likely to have dry eyes, and are more prone to lens film and deposits, which increase the risk of infective conjunctivitis and corneal ulcers. Many of the corneal ulcers are sterile, and with a co-operative patient, who seeks advice early, corneal ulceration should not be a particular problem. Should an infected corneal ulcer with an anterior uveitis occur, it is inadvisable for the patient to wear extended wear soft lenses again.

If it is possible to regain binocular vision with spectacles this should be done; the alternative being a secondary intraocular lens implant. Superficial corneal neovascularization (and occasionally deep) is more liable to occur in older than in younger extended wear wearers, and is liable to progress much further. More neovascularization is tolerated in aphakics, as there is often no other alternative to their extended wear lens. It may be reduced by using a high water content lens, which is as thin as possible. An intracorneal haemorrhage may occur in aphakic patients wearing EW soft lenses (Laroche and Campbell, 1987). We have had two such cases in the last 12 years, with complete resolution within a week (Figure 11.7). A further serious complication which may occur from the use of both rigid and soft lenses, is an aphakic endophthalmitis in the presence of a filtering bleb resulting from the surgery (Bellows and McCulley, 1981).

Difficulties can occur when patients move away from the area of the practice, when it may be difficult to arrange for them to see a local ophthalmologist if they have problems. There is also the problem of elderly patients being unable to travel at times due to illness, and of not taking notice of the danger signal of a red eye (Figure 11.8 and 11.9). When these situations occur the cessation of extended wear soft lenses must be considered. It is particularly for aphakic patients that reasonably priced disposable lenses are needed, as it is often impossible to remove deposits satisfactorily from a soft lens, and new lenses are frequently needed.

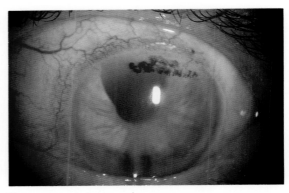

Figure 11.7 Aphakic patient wearing a soft lens, with an intracorneal haemorrhage

Lenses for infants and children

Infants and young children may need to be fitted with contact lenses to correct unilateral and bilateral aphakia, anisometropia, high myopia, accommodative convergent squint, and for unilateral occlusion. They usually manage very well with contact lenses, but it depends not only on the child's co-operation, but also on the attitude of the parents. Extended wear soft lenses are usually the most suitable, for the very young initially, but there are now high RGP lenses, which may be worn for extended wear. Silicone lenses have been used extensively in North America but extended wear soft lenses are chiefly preferred in the UK. Daily wear soft lenses have been used more recently, when it has been possible for a patient to insert and remove lenses. As the commonest reason for fitting contact lenses is for aphakia, it will be discussed in detail.

For congenital cataracts, it is essential that they are operated on as soon as possible after birth (Taylor *et al.*, 1979). The first eye is usually operated on at about six weeks from birth, or as soon as possible after this; and the second eye a week or so later. Correction of the aphakia with an extended wear soft lens should be started very soon after each operation. The lenses can be difficult to insert, as there is a tendency for them to fold, and bubbles may form under the lens, causing the lens to be ejected as the lids are closed. The infant needs to be restrained while lying down, by wrapping them in a blanket or sheet, to hold the arms to the body.

If there is difficulty inserting the lens due to marked blepharospasm, one more lid retractors may need to be used. Most infants will co-operate better after several visits, and it should soon be possible to insert and remove lenses without any problem. It is essential that the mother, or another relative, is taught to insert and remove lenses as soon as possible, but this may take time. Fitting of the lenses is now discussed.

Extended wear soft lenses

High water content lenses should be used, as these can be thicker, and will correct more astigmatism. Initially, lenses were fitted from keratometry done under a general anaesthetic. From these findings it is now not necessary to do this measurement, as the BOZR required has been found to be fairly consistent with age. A suggested fitting set of EW soft lenses for infantile aphakia would have a TD of 13 mm, BOZRs of 7.5 and 7.8 mm, and each radius in powers of +20.0, +25.0, +30.0 and +35.0 DS. For an aphakic infant from one to three months old, a lens with a 7.50 mm BOZR, 13 mm TD and power of about +30.0 to +35.0 DS is fitted initially. In the case of a smaller than usual eye, a slightly steeper fit and smaller TD may be required. The fit may be

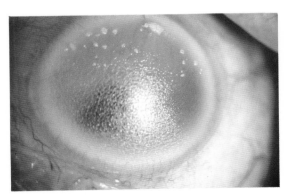

Figure 11.8 Aphakic patient wearing an extended wear soft lens, who could not be located, and had not seen an ophthalmologist for over a year

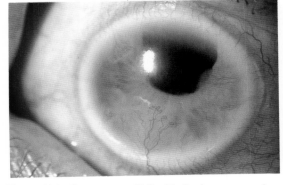

Figure 11.9 Same eye as 11.8 with the lens removed. Apart from some neovascularization the cornea was clear

checked by observing the movement of the lens on the eye, which should be at least 1.0 mm. Provided the fit is satisfactory, the power can be checked by retinoscopy, and changed if necessary. The lens should be over corrected by +2.0 to +3.0 dioptres, as an infant or very young child is mainly using its near vision. It may be possible to insert a lens at the end of the operation, but most ophthalmologists prefer to do this a few days later. Checks on the lens should be done at 24 hours, one to two weeks, one month, and then at about two-monthly intervals, or at any time should there be a problem. A spare lens should be kept available, and one also given to the parents, so that they can insert a new lens should a lens be broken or lost. It should be stressed to the parents that the child must always be wearing a lens. As the child's eye grows it will probably be necessary for the fit of the lens to be flattened to 7.8 mm BOZR by the age of a year or so. Further flattening may be needed after the age of two or three years. For unilateral aphakia, after fitting the aphakic eye with a contact lens, the phakic eye must initially be occluded to make sure that the child uses the aphakic eye, to prevent amblyopia. Most children prefer an occluding lens either as glasses or a contact lens on the phakic eye, rather than patching. Close watch must be kept on both the fit and the power of the lens, the latter by means of retinoscopy, while the child is growing. When the child starts to take an interest in more distant vision, the lens power should be adjusted for this, and bifocal glasses given to correct any residual astigmatism, together with the near vision correction for the aphakic eye or eyes.

Children with bilateral aphakia can do well with contact lenses, but can also do well with glasses. If contact lens correction is used, glasses should also be prescribed, for use when contact lens wear is not possible.

Rigid gas-permeable lenses

These are more difficult to fit, and are more suitable for children aged two or three years old and above. They may be used on a daily wear basis, but high *Dk* lenses are suitable for extended wear, as are silicone lenses (Harris, 1985). It may be possible to do a keratometry on the child, so that the lenses are fitted in the usual way. High *Dk*

EW lenses must be fitted about 0.05–0.10 mm flatter than the flattest keratometer reading. If these lenses are fitted too tight a lens adhesion problem may occur, and the lens be difficult to remove. When this happens, liberal use of N-saline solution should aid removal. If keratometry readings are not possible then trial lenses should be used, and the fit assessed by the fluorescein pattern and lens movement. For children below two years a starting lens should be about 7.5 mm BOZR, a 7.7 mm BOZR for ages two to four years, and a 7.9 mm BOZR above the age of four years. The fluorescein pattern should show a very light central corneal touch, and should never be apex clear. The lens loss and complication rates tend to be lower with rigid lenses than with soft EW lenses (Pe'er *et al.*, 1987).

Occlusion treatment

This is necessary for conditions such as unilateral aphakia, and as treatment for amblyopia when the dominant eye is occluded. This can be conveniently done by patching, either directly on the skin, or on glasses. Some children will not tolerate an eye patch, so an occlusive spectacle or contact lens can be tried, usually of high plus power. Soft contact lenses can either be a high plus power, or else may have a dense black tint to cover the whole lens, or just large enough to cover the pupil.

Other indications

When a child is unwilling to wear glasses for high myopia, or moderate hypermetropia, contact lenses may be acceptable. This is particularly applicable with an accommodative convergent squint.

Complications of lens wear in infants and children

The parents must be provided with full and comprehensive written instructions regarding the handling of the lenses, and what symptoms to look out for. It is most important to remove a lens immediately if there are problems, and for the

child to be seen by an ophthalmologist as soon as possible.

The main problems are lens loss and breakage, which are usually caused by rubbing the eyes. Spare lenses should always be kept in stock, as lens loss can be a frequent problem for infants and children. Infants usually tolerate lenses well for the first year or two, but it is common for periods of being unco-operative to occur immediately following the second year. Lens contamination by surface film or deposits requires a change of lens. A lens must be removed immediately should discharge, redness or pain occur in the eye, or if a white spot is noticed on the cornea, which might indicate a corneal ulcer.

References

Aphakia

BELLOWS, A.R. and MCCULLEY, J.P. (1981) Endophthalmitis in aphakic patients with unplanned filtering blebs wearing contact lenses. *Ophthalmology*, **88**, 839–843

LAROCHE, R.R. and CAMPBELL, R.C. (1987) Intracorneal haemorrhage induced by chronic extended wear of a soft contact lens. *The CLAO Journal*, **13**, 39–40

Further reading

Aphakia

BERGER, R.D. and STREATEN, B.W. (1981) Fungal growth in aphakic soft contact lenses. *American Journal of Ophthalmology*, **91**, 630–633

EICHENBAUM, J.W., FELDSTEIN, M. and PODOS, S.M. (1982) Extended wear aphakic soft contact lenses and corneal ulcers. *British Journal of Opthalmology*, **66**, 663–666

ING, M.R. (1981) Experience with extended wear hydrogel lenses for aphakia. *Annals of Ophthalmology*, **13**, 181–182

KERSLEY, H.J. (1977) Contact lenses in aphakia. *Transactions of the Ophthalmological Societies of the United Kingdom*, **97**, 142–144

KERSLEY, H.J. (1985) Contact lens management of aphakia. In *Cataract Surgery*, (eds A.D. McG. Steele and R.C. Drews), Butterworths, London, pp. 197–212

LEMBACH, R.G. and KEATES, R.H. (1984) Long term follow up of extended wear Aphakic Permalenses. *The CLAO Journal*, **10**, 83–87

MARTIN, N.F., KRACHER, G.P., STARK, W.J., *et al.* (1983) Extended wear soft contact lenses for aphakic correction. *Archives of Ophthalmology*, **101**, 39–41

MATSUDA, M., INABA, M., SUDA, T., and MACRAE, S.M. (1988) Corneal endothelial changes associated with aphakic extended contact lens wear. *Archives of Ophthalmology*, **106**, 70–72

SALZ, J.J. and SCHLANGER, J.L. (1983) Complications of aphakic extended wear lenses encountered during a seven year period in 100 eyes. *The CLAO Journal*, **91**, 241–244

STEIN, H.A. and SLATT, B. (1974) Contact lenses after cataract surgery: A review of 200 aphakic patients fitted with soft lenses. *Canadian Journal of Ophthalmology*, **9**, 79–83

STEIN, H.A. (1981) Aphakic selection for contact lenses, intraocular lenses spectacles. Review of 1,000 cataract operations. *Contact and Intraocular Lens Medical Journal*, **7**, 210–218

TANDON, M.K., DAVIES, M.S., WISHART, D. *et al.* (1981) Extended wear soft contact lenses in the correction of aphakia. *Transactions of the Ophthalmological Societies of the United Kingdom*, **101**, 65–68

WEIS, D.R. (1982) Long term results of wearing hard contact lenses in monocular aphakia. *Ophthalmology*, **89**, 1003–1005

References

Infants and children

HARRIS, M. (1985) Correction of pediatric aphakia with silicone contact lenses. *The CLAO Journal*, **11**, 343–347

PE'ER, J., ROSE, L., COHEN, E. and BEN EZRA, D. (1987) Hard and soft contact fitting in infants. *The CLAO Journal*, **13**, 46–49

TAYLOR, D., VAEGAN, J.A., MORRIS, J., *et al.* (1979) Amblyopia in bilateral infantile and juvenile cataract. *Transactions of the Ophthalmological Societies of the United Kingdom*, **99**, 170–176

Further reading

Infants and children

ARFFA, R.C., MARVELLI, T.L. and MORGAN, T.S. (1985) Keratometric and refractive results in pediatric aphakia. *Archives of Ophthalmology*, **103**, 1656–1659

CUTTER, S.I., NELSON, L.B. and CALHAN, J.H. (1985) Extended wear contact lenses in paediatric aphakia. *Journal of Paediatric Ophthalmology and Strabismus*, **22**, 86–91

DAVIS, P.P. and TARBUCK, D.H.J. (1977) Management of cataracts in infancy and childhood. *Transactions of the Ophthalmological Society of the United Kingdom*, **97**, 148–152

GURLAN, J. (1979) Use of silicone lenses in infants and children. *Ophthalmology*, **86**, 1599–1604

NELSON, L.B., CUTLER, S.I., CALHOUN, J.H., *et al.* (1985) Silsoft extended wear contact lenses in pediatric aphakia. *Opthalmology*, **92**, 1529–1531

PRATT-JOHNSON, I.A. and TILLSON, G. (1985) Hard contacts in the management of congenital cataracts. *Journal of Pediatric Ophthalmology and Strabismus*, **22**, 94–96

ROGERS, G.L. (1980) Extended wear silicone lenses in children with cataracts. *Ophthalmology*, **87**, 867–870

SAUNDERS, R.A., and ELLIS, F.D. (1981) Empirical fitting of hard contact lenses in infants and young children. *Ophthalmology*, **88**, 127–130

SPEEDWELL, L. (1987) Contact lens fitting in infants and pre-school children. *The Optician*, September 4, 26–39

WEISSMAN, B. (1983) Fitting aphakic children with contact lenses. *Journal of the American Optometric Association*, **54**, 235–237

12

Contact lenses for keratoconus and after corneal surgery

Keratoconus is a thinning of the cornea with progressive, conical ectasia. It is usually bilateral, appearing during the second decade, and often occurring in one eye initially. There is a tendency for it to progress for several years before stabilizing in the fourth decade. When advanced, there are three main types of cone:

1. Round or nipple-shaped cone, which is commonest.
2. Oval or sagging cone.
3. Large globus cone.

The round cone is a central, or just below centre, usually steep protrusion, and less than 5 mm in diameter. The oval cone usually lies in the lower temporal quadrant and is about 5–6 mm in diameter, while the globus cone can be up to three quarters of the corneal surface.

Cone size can be determined by photodiagnosis (Shaw, Sewell and Gasset, 1973). The cone image is viewed against the red fundus reflex, with the pupil dilated, using a direct ophthalmoscope and a high plus lens at about 50 cm. The size, shape, and location of the conical area can be determined. The original method was to photograph the red reflex.

Keratoconus seems to be more prevalent in males. Reports that it may be caused by wearing rigid corneal lenses, or that contact lenses can stop or slow down the progression of the cone, are unsubstantiated.

Diagnosis of keratoconus

1. Increasing irregular astigmatism, with alteration of the cylinder axes, usually in an oblique direction.

2. Swirling, 'scissors' movement with retinoscopy.
3. Vision not correctable to 6/6 with spectacles.
4. Keratometry shows distortion and inclination of the mires, with steep readings.
5. Distortion of the circular mires of a Placido disc, or the photokeratoscope.
6. Slit-lamp examination of the cornea to show a Fleischers pigment ring at the base of the cone, visible nerve fibres, deep stromal vertical striae, and apical corneal thinning and scarring.

Classification of keratoconus

1. Early – mean K readings flatter than 6.80 mm.
2. Advanced – mean K readings between 6.80 and 6.00 mm.
3. Severe – mean K readings steeper than 6.00 mm.

Visual correction in keratoconus

In the early stages of keratoconus, the vision may be adequately corrected by spectacles, which should be used for as long as the vision remains satisfactory.

Gasset (1975) has described a method for determining the starting point for refraction when retinoscopy is not possible. The best possible keratometry measurement is done, and it is assumed that the normal dioptric power of the cornea is about 43.00 DS. Any increase in this by the K

readings will be the amount of sphero cylindrical refraction.

When spectacles no longer give adequate vision, contact lenses should be tried. A PMMA lens gives better vision by substituting its spherical front surface, for the toric front surface of the cornea. The correction of keratoconus is a great challenge, in order to fit a comfortable lens which gives good vision.

Rigid lens fitting

Note the position, shape and diameter of the cone, which can be estimated by photodiagnosis, or from a Fleischer ring if present. Any apical scaring may reduce visual improvement. The apex of the cone is normally below the visual axis, which can produce a loose fitting lens. Ideally the lens should fit with light apical touch, and mid-peripheral touch. What is described as a three point touch is a good general guideline (Figure 12.1). A mid-peripheral touch which extends around the whole lens periphery should be avoided as it prevents adequate venting under the lens. There should be a small edge uplift below, which is surprisingly well tolerated by the lower lid margin.

Keratometry measurements are done, which may be difficult due to distortion of the mires. An automatic keratometer is unlikely to give a reading in advanced keratoconus. The range of the keratometer can be extended as described in Chapter 5.

Spherical PMMA lenses

Typical PMMA trial lenses are spherical well blended tri-curves with a BOZD of 7.0 mm and two peripheral curves 1 mm and 3 mm flatter than the BOZR. The first BPZD is 7.80 mm and the TD 8.40 mm (Table A8.7 in Appendix 8). These lenses will provide a starting point in assessing the fit of the lens on the eye by its fluorescein pattern. The initial lens should have a BOZR the mean of the two K readings. The BOZR should be changed so that there is about 2 mm of light apical touch, which still allows a thin film of tears to pass over the corneal apex on blinking. Too much apical clearance will cause heavy peripheral touch, preventing adequate venting under the lens. If the lens is too large for the cone as seen by heavy peripheral touch, the TD should be reduced e.g. to 8.0 mm, and BOZD to 6.5 mm. It may then be necessary to steepen the BOZR to maintain a 2 mm light apical touch. If the lens is too small for the cone the fluorescein pattern will show a 3–4 mm area of apical touch, and a larger 9 mm lens should give a better fit, with the same BOZR.

On over refraction to assess the final power of the lens, many patients may have some residual astigmatism, which can be put into spectacles to wear on top of the contact lenses.

The McGuire keratoconus trial lenses comprise three sets: one each for nipple, oval and globus cones. They vary in overall diameter, and have four well blended peripheral curves (Caroline, McGuire and Doughman, 1978).

Aspheric rigid gas-permeable lenses

RGP lenses are ideally suited for keratoconus because of their good oxygen transmissibility and thermal conductivity. As the lens tends to flex on the eye, the vision may not be as good with a PMMA lens, but should be more comfortable (Maguen *et al.*, 1983).

Caroline and Norman in an as yet unpublished paper, have described the use of RGP lenses with a central spherical zone, and an aspheric intermediate zone to correct keratoconus. The trial lenses have BOZDs from 6.4–7.4 mm as the BOZR goes from 6.4–8.6 mm, and TDs varying from 9.2–10.0 mm. By photokeratoscopy Caroline and Norman found that the cornea above the midline remains

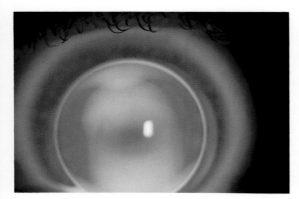

Figure 12.1 Keratoconus patient with 'three point touch' rigid corneal lens

relatively normal in curvature in early keratoconus. The inferior cornea invaginates below the cone, which increases the appearance of corneal protrusion. They think that the curvature of the superior cornea is the important fitting consideration. Measurements may be made by photokeratoscopy or by taking upper paracentral readings with a keratometer. A trial lens with a BOZR of the flattest superior corneal reading obtained is used. If neither of these measurements is available, trial lenses can be used to evaluate the fit. The lens should stabilize slightly high on the cornea, and the optic zone should have about 2–4 mm of light apical touch. There will be some edge lift below, and this must not be decreased, or the superior fit will be made tighter. The TD is made 2.0 mm smaller than the horizontal visible iris diameter (HVID). An over refraction will give the final lens power required.

Ciba Vision produce a CAB lens with a bi-elliptical back surface, the Persecon E Keratoconus (PEK) lens, which allows the lens pressure to be spread over a large area (Astin, 1987). Table A8.8 in Appendix 8 gives the parameters of the trial lenses. The 9.30 mm TD lens is suitable for most corneas, but the larger 9.80 mm lens may be better when the smaller lens is unstable, and with a large globus cone. The aim is a light apical touch at the centre of the lens to ensure good pressure distribution. In changing from a 9.30 to a 9.80 TD, a 0.20 mm flatter BOZR should be used, and vice versa. The lens should move smoothly on the eye with blinking, and is usually a comfortable lens to wear.

Advanced and severe keratoconus

In advanced keratoconus a high minus lens power is required, which entails a thick edge to the lens. To improve matters, the power required can be divided between the hard lens, and either spectacles, or a soft lens using the piggyback method (see below).

When an advanced cone requires refitting, a smaller steeper lens may be needed. This may cause problems with discomfort, if the lens is felt more by the lid margins on blinking.

Advanced and severe nipple cone

To fit an advanced or severe nipple cone, McGuire nipple cone lenses may be used. These have an 8.1 mm TD, 5.5 mm BOZD, and four peripheral curves. The BOZR is altered to give 2 mm of light apical touch. Bubbles may appear under the lens at the base of the cone, and they can be removed by flattening the BOZR or decreasing the BOZD (Caroline, McGuire and Doughman, 1978).

An alternative is to try a 9.5 mm TD lens, with an 8.10 mm BOZD, which produces a larger area of heavy apical touch.

Advanced and severe oval cone and globus cone

The McGuire oval cone lenses have a TD of 8.6 mm, a BOZD of 6 mm and four peripheral curves. The aim is a 2 mm light apical touch.

The McGuire globus cone lenses have a TD of 9.1 mm, a BOZD of 6.5 mm and four peripheral curves.

Adjustments to oval and globus lenses, are made in the same way as for the nipple cone lenses by:

1. Adjusting the BOZD to fit the cone diameter.
2. Adjusting the BOZR to give 2 mm of light apical touch.
3. Adjusting the peripheral curves to the underlying corneal curvature.

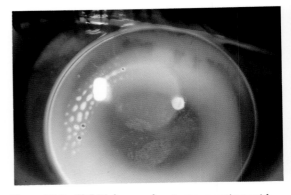

Figure 12.2 PMMA lens on keratoconus patient with 'heavy' central touch with corneal abrasions, and a paracentral fenestration hole with bubble impressions around the periphery

Keratoconus patients wearing PMMA or RGP lenses need to be seen about every six months, to assess the fit and check for corneal oedema, abrasions and scarring (Figure 12.2).

Soft contact lenses

When a patient is unable to tolerate any kind of rigid lens, it is worthwhile trying a soft lens. It should be more comfortable, and may give surprisingly good vision, particularly when worn with spectacles to correct any residual astigmatism. By increasing the centre thickness of a middle water content lens e.g. 55–70%, to not less than 0.35 mm and up to 0.55 mm depending on the power, more astigmatism will be corrected. The lens should be fitted flat and the BOZR about 7.8 –8.4 mm, with a total diameter between 13.5–14.5 mm, to give good stability (Gasset, 1972).

The tri-curve soft Flexlens

The soft tri-curve Flexlens is specially designed for keratoconus, with a centre thickness of 0.55 mm and is made in the USA. The trial set has BOZRs from 6.25 to 8.5 mm, TDs of 14.0 to 14.5 mm and a FOZD of 8 mm. The BOZR fits the corneal apex, and a total diameter about 3 mm larger than the cornea. It is manufactured in a wide range of powers and parameters. It works best with the round, nipple type cone, and not so well on the larger and sagging cones. Glasses may be required on top to correct any residual astigmatism.

Trapezoidal soft lenses

Ruben (1978) has designed a soft lens with a flat BOZR of 11–15 mm and a steeper back peripheral curve of 8.5 mm and a TD of 15 mm. On the eye, the eye and lens both mould to each other, so that cornea tends to flatten, and the BOZR steepens.

Bausch and Lomb 'C' series soft lens

This is useful for the correction of keratoconus with large round cones, in the higher myopic

powers. The lenses are spun cast, with an TD of 13.50 mm, and have a small optic zone.

Combination or 'piggyback' lenses

A soft lens alone may not give satisfactory vision, and a hard lens may be unstable and uncomfortable. The instability is due both to the irregular corneal curvature, and to the thick edge of the high minus power lens, which is necessary to correct the vision. To overcome the problem of the lens edge thickness, the necessary power can be divided between the contact lens, and spectacles which are worn on top. However, many patients do not wish to wear glasses on top of their contact lenses, and a combination of a soft contact lens with an RGP lens fitted on top may be tried. This was first described by Westerhout (1973). The term 'piggyback' lens is used for this method. The rigid lens can either be free on the soft lens surface, or may fit into a circular cut out portion, in the centre of the front surface of the soft lens (Figure 12.3).

The soft lens will produce a more regular front surface than the cornea, and thus make the rigid lens fit more stable. When the rigid lens is used on the front surface of the soft lens, the latter should be made of a low to middle water content material,

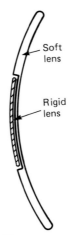

Figure 12.3 A 'piggyback' rigid corneal lens fitting into the centre of a soft lens

e.g. 38–45%. With the soft lens on the eye, a K reading of the front of the lens will be a guide to the rigid lens fitting. For the insert method, the central cut out portion needs to be about 8.5 mm in diameter, about 0.2 mm deep and the soft lens material in the middle range of water content i.e. 45–55%. The RGP lens should be about 0.2–0.3 mm smaller in overall diameter than the cut out diameter in the soft lens (Caroline and Doughman, 1979). The RGP lens should be of the highest gas permeability that is available, to allow maximum passage of oxygen to the cornea. Ideally not too much minus power should be put on the RGP lens, and the remainder should go on the soft lens.

If the RGP lens is easily dislodged from the soft lens by the upper lid, the high minus RGP lens can be fitted over a high plus soft lens. This is most useful for when the cornea is flat, e.g. after keratoplasty. The piggyback system can give good visual results, and be very comfortable, but some patients find it inconvenient to manage the two different types of lenses.

Scleral lenses

Scleral lenses are now only used for patients who cannot obtain adequate vision with any other kind of contact lens, and who do not wish to have surgery. Methods of fitting scleral lenses are covered in Chapter 13. There are still a few patients in the UK, who are wearing scleral lenses, with good visual results, but with poor wearing times. However, in the future it may be possible to make scleral lenses from a high gas permeable material, which should give improved wearing times (Pullum, 1987).

Rigid/soft contact lens

The Saturn II lens, now made by Pilkington Barnes Hind is a RGP lens (*Dk* 14 at 35°C) with a surrounding soft lens skirt, with a water content of 25% (Figure 12.3). The BOZRs are 7.2 to 8.2 mm, BOZD 8 mm, TD 14.3 mm and powers from +6.0 to −13.0 DS. There has been a problem with the rigid/soft junction, but an improved

design should be available in the USA soon (Figure 12.4). The lens is fitted with regard to the rigid lens in the usual way.

Two points need to be made about keratoconus patients. Firstly, many patients have an increased corneal apical sensitivity during early keratoconus, which usually becomes reduced as the cone increases. Ruben (1978) has suggested severing corneal nerves with a trephine, but the effect is not permanent. Secondly, as the keratoconus progresses, the patients become increasingly dependent on contact lenses, which can produce psychological problems for them. It is particularly important to be sympathetic when dealing with these patients, and to remember their predicament. When rigid or soft lenses are no longer comfortable, or the vision inadequate because of a severe cone or corneal scarring, a penetrating keratoplasty may be indicated.

Contact lens fitting after keratoplasty

It is estimated that up to 25% of patients will need a contact lens to obtain improved vision after keratoplasty. As well as these lenses, many patients may require a therapeutic lens to protect the graft surface, and this is dealt with in Chapter 14.

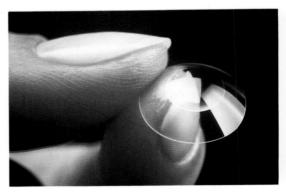

Figure 12.4   A Saturn II soft lens with an RGP centre (Courtesy of Pilkington Barnes Hind)

To improve the vision, the choice of lens will depend on the amount of astigmatism. A daily wear soft lens can be tried if the amount of astigmatism is under 2.50 D, but spectacles may also give adequate vision (Mannis, 1986). For astigmatism greater than 2.5 D an RGP lens is needed (Grenvert *et al.*, 1985). If the astigmatism is very high, a back toric rigid lens may be tried, or else the 'piggyback method' of a rigid lens on top of a soft one. For the majority of cases an RGP lens should give the best vision.

Fitting the phakic patient

The amount of corneal astigmatism present will usually require an RGP lens. The lens is best fitted after all sutures have been removed, which is generally about a year after the operation. The lens should centre well, have adequate movement, give good vision, and be comfortable. The lens can be fitted inside the graft, but it is usually preferable to fit it larger than the graft, as a 9.0 mm tricurve RGP lens. For high astigmatism, and when there is too much edge lift below, try a steeper and/or smaller lens.

For insufficient movement, i.e. less than 1.5 mm, try a smaller and/or flatter lens. Finally, if the lens decentres too much, or the movement is excessive and unstable, a larger and/or steeper lens can be tried. If all attempts to fit a rigid lens are unsuccessful, then a daily wear soft lens can be tried as below.

Fitting the aphakic patient

If able to handle lenses, the aphakic patient can be fitted with either daily wear soft, or RGP lenses. Daily wear soft lenses of moderate water content i.e. 45–55%, can correct several dioptres of astigmatism due to their thickness. It is important to watch carefully for any vascularization of the graft, which will need a looser fitting lens. Should the vascularization continue, soft lens wear should be stopped, and a change made to an RGP lens.

If a patient is not able to handle a contact lens, an extended wear soft lens will be required (Dangle *et al.*, 1983). A high water content lens should be used, and fitted as loose as possible.

Vascularization of the graft is much more common in extended wear patients, and may require cessation of lens wear altogether, if the patient cannot handle a lens themselves. With any kind of soft lens, any residual astigmatism can be put in bifocal spectacles, as the patient will need a reading correction to wear on top anyway.

Possible reasons for discontinuing the lenses are:

1. Graft rejection, which is more likely to occur with rigid lenses. The graft usually clears when the lens is stopped, and it is sometimes possible to resume contact lens wear.
2. Inadequate vision usually occurs from an unstable rigid lens. A change to a daily wear soft lens, and spectacles can be tried.
3. Vascularization of the graft is commonest in extended wear soft lens patients.
4. Lens intolerance may occur in rigid lens wearers.
5. Corneal ulcers are a serious complication, which may require cessation of lens wear, if there is a definite risk of recurrence.

Contact lens fitting after radial keratotomy

It is said that 40–60% of patients who undergo a radial keratotomy for myopia are as much as 1.0 D or more from ametropia (Arrowsmith and Marks, 1984; Sawelson and Marks, 1983).

Approximately 4% of patients undergoing radial keratotomy will need to wear contact lenses to obtain satisfactory vision (Shivitz *et al.*, 1986). The central cornea will be flat, with a steeper periphery. It is best to wait for at least three months following the operation before fitting a lens. As soft contact lenses can produce superficial neovascularization related to the corneal incisions, an RGP lens is preferable. The initial trial lens should have a BOZR the same as the flattest preoperative reading, and a TD about 9.5 mm. The BOZR and/or TD are altered to give the best possible fit. The lens will have a thick pool of tears and air bubbles under its centre, and a single 0.3 mm fenestration is often required to relieve discomfort. The lens power will probably be about the same as the original myopia, due to the plus

tear lens. In one series no corneal neovascularization was found with RGP lens wear (Shivitz *et al.*, 1986). Many patients who could not wear a rigid contact lens before the operation, can manage to wear one afterwards, presumably due to diminished corneal sensitivity.

Should it not be possible to fit an RGP lens successfully, a daily wear soft lens should be tried, and not an extended wear soft lens, due to the increased incidence of corneal neovascularization with the latter. The BOZR of the first trial soft lens is again based on the preoperative keratometry reading. A soft lens can produce the tight lens syndrome if fitted too tightly. The corneal curvature can become steeper from corneal oedema, so that patients wearing soft lenses must be watched for any alteration in corneal curvature. Other complications are corneal neovascularization and infection, particularly by *Pseudomonas*, of the incisions sites. As for any scarred cornea, recurrent erosions may occur around the incision sites, particularly when rigid lenses are used.

References

ARROWSMITH, P.N. and MARKS, R.G. (1984) Visual, refractive, and keratometric results of radial keratotomy: one year follow up. *Archives of Ophthalmology*, **102**, 1617–1618

ASTIN, C. (1987) Bi-elliptical contact lenses for keratoconus. *The Journal of the British Contact Lens Association*, **10**, 24–28

CAROLINE, P.J. and DOUGHMAN, D.J. (1979) A new piggyback lens design for correction of irregular astigmatism. *Contact and Intraocular Lens Medical Journal*, **5**, 40–44

CAROLINE, P.J., McGUIRE, J.R. and DOUGHMAN, D.J. (1978) A new contact lens design for keratoconus – a continuing report. *Contact and Intraocular Lens Medical Journal*, **4**, 69–73

DANGLE, M.E., KRACHER, G.P., START, W.J., *et al.* (1983) Aphakic extended wear contact lenses after penetrating keratoplasty. *American Journal of Ophthalmology*, **95**, 156–160

GASSET, A.R. (1972) Hydrophilic contact lenses in the management of keratoconus. *Journal of the American Optometric Association*, **43**, 338–341

GASSET, A.R. (1975) Simplified refracting techniques in keratoconus. *Annals of Ophthalmology*, **7**, 117–121

GRENVERT, G., COHEN, F.J., ARENTSEN, J.J., *et al.* (1985) Fitting gas permeable contact lenses after penetrating keratoplasty. *American Journal of Ophthalmology*, **99**, 511–514

MAGUEN, E., ESPINOSA, G., ROSNER, R. and NESBURN, A.B. (1983) Long term wear of Polycon lenses in keratoconus. *The CLAO Journal*, **9**, 57–59

MANNIS, M.J. (1986) Indications for Contact Lens Fitting after Keratoplasty. *The CLAO Journal*, **12**, 225–228

PULLUM K.W. (1987) Feasibility study for the production of gas permeable scleral lenses using ocular impression techniques. *Transaction of the British Contact Lens Association Annual Clinical Conference No. 4*, 35–39

RUBEN, M. (ed.) (1978) Correction of keratoconus with soft lenses. In *Soft Contact Lenses: Clinical and Applied Technology*, Bailliere Tindall, London, pp. 256–260

SAWELSON, H.R. and MARKS, R.G. (1983) Two years results of radial keratotomy. *Archives of Ophthalmology*, **103**, 505–510

SHAW, E.L., SEWELL, J. and GASSET, A.R. (1973) Photodiagnosis of keratoconus. *Annals of Ophthalmology*, **5**, 297–300

SHIVITZ, I.A., RUSSELL, B.M., ARROWSMITH, B.N. and MARKS, B.D. (1986) Optical correction of post-operative radial keratotomy patients with contact lenses. *The CLAO Journal*, **12**, 59–62

WESTERHOUT, D. (1973) The combination lens. *The Contact Lens*, **4**, 3–9

Further reading

INSLER, M.S. and COOPER, H.D. (1986) New correlations in keratoconus using pachymetric and keratometric analysis. *The CLAO Journal*, **12**, 101–105

KORB, D.R. (1984) Recent developments in fitting contact lenses for keratoconus. *Journal of American Optometric Association*, **55**, 172–174

MANABE, R., MATSUDA, M. and SUDA, T. (1986) Photokeratoscopy in fitting contact lenses after penetrating keratoplasty. *British Journal of Opthalmology*, **70**, 55–59

WEISSMAN, B. and HOFFBAUER, J. (1982) Fitting contact lenses following corneal transplantation. *Optometric Monthly*, **73**, 562–565

13

Rigid scleral and coloured contact lenses

PMMA scleral contact lenses

PMMA scleral lenses were formerly called haptic lenses in the UK since the term was first used by Dallos in 1936. For several decades prior to the 1930s, the lenses were made of blown glass, and then of solid ground glass. In the 1940s PMMA superseded glass in the manufacture of scleral lenses, as it was lighter in weight, less expensive and easier to manufacture. Patients who have worn glass scleral lenses are often not so comfortable with PMMA lenses made to the same specifications. Scleral lenses are difficult to fit and to wear, and there are now very few ophthalmologists who have ever fitted them. They were used to correct refractive errors, and in particular to improve the poor vision due to corneal irregularity. The use of scleral lenses has decreased since the advent of soft contact lenses, because the latter are better for most of the therapeutic reasons for which scleral lenses were formerly used. However, in the UK there are still some patients wearing scleral lenses for conditions such as myopia, keratoconus, high astigmatism and corneal scarring, and who do not wish to change to rigid corneal or soft lenses.

Indications for scleral lenses

1. Sports e.g. competitive swimming and diving.
2. When a patient wishes to have a new scleral lens.
3. To incorporate a horizontal or base up prism in the optical correction.
4. Some cases of keratoconus, where soft, rigid corneal or rigid/soft lenses are unsuitable, and a corneal graft is contra-indicated.
5. For splinting, e.g. following keratoplasty, where tilting of the graft has occurred (Figure 13.1), and to correct ptosis (see below).
6. As a prosthetic shell or artificial eye. Due to the lens thickness it is possible to simulate an anterior chamber. Lack of this is often a reason for a patient rejecting a cosmetic rigid corneal, or soft contact lenses.

General principles of scleral lens fitting

A scleral lens can be divided into:

1. A central corneal part (or optic), which must have adequate corneal clearance to allow an even flow of tears over the cornea.

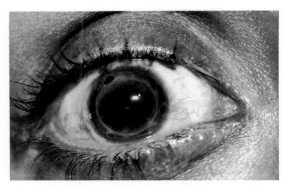

Figure 13.1 Scleral lens wearer with 9 dioptres of astigmatism following a keratoplasty for keratoconus (Courtesy of Professor E G Woodward)

2. A surrounding scleral part which must be in apposition to the globe, and the weight spread evenly, to support the optic accurately in its correct position (Figure 13.2).
3. The transition between the two, which overlies the limbus. Tear interchange under the lens may be by a fenestration hole, usually at the temporal limbus (Figure 13.2), or by channels or grooves under the lens (Figure 13.3). The aim is to produce a lens which can be worn comfortably for as long as necessary.

Scleral lens fitting

Scleral lenses may be made by taking an impression of the eye, and pressing a shell from the plaster cast obtained from the impression.

Alternatively they may be fitted by the preformed lens method, which entails fitting from trial lenses. Both methods are used and will be briefly described.

Impression method

With the patient in a comfortable reclined position, the eye is anaesthetized using local anaesthetic drops with adrenaline. A fixation object such as a light, is then positioned for the other eye to look at, so that the eye to be moulded is looking slightly nasally from the straight ahead position. An appropriate sized scleral injection shell with a hollow stem (Figure 13.4) is placed on the eye, and an alginate impression material such as Kromopan or Moldite which has been freshly mixed, is slowly injected down the stem with a syringe. The shell should be gently pulled away from the globe while

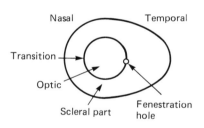

Figure 13.2 Scleral contact lens with fenestration hole

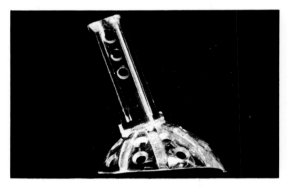

Figure 13.4 Scleral injection shell

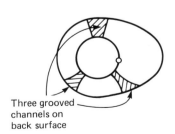

Figure 13.3 Scleral contact lens with grooved channels

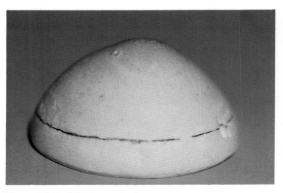

Figure 13.5 Plaster cast of an eye

this is done, and then allowed to sink back onto the globe again, in order to avoid bubbles and thin areas in the cast. The shell has several holes through which the impression material penetrates, and as it sets the impression is secured to the shell. The patient must keep their other eye still in the fixation position, while the impression material sets, which usually takes about 2–3 minutes, depending on the mixture and the room temperature. The shell is then gently removed from the eye, and a plaster cast made from the impression obtained (Figure 13.5). Alternatively an insertion shell, with either a small solid handle, or which is manipulated with a suction holder may be used, and the impression material is placed in the shell prior to placing it on the eye.

A plastic shell is then made by gently heating a square of Perspex (PMMA) about 1 mm thick, and pressing it over the plaster cast. When cool the shell is removed, and the excess Perspex cut away.

The edges of the shell are shaped, rounded and polished, and the limbus is marked out on the shell, with the shell on the cast. The lens is fenestrated with a 1 mm hole at the temporal limbus or channelled, to allow tear interchange, and the transition area ground out to give limbal clearance. The back optic radius is then ground out on the lens, and the front surface ground to give the required refraction. The lens is then checked on the patient's eye using fluorescein, to note the corneal clearance, and the size and movement of the bubble (Figures 13.6 and 13.7). Localized vessel blanching will indicate an excessive touch over the sclera. Either the scleral or optic parts may be ground out to give the appropriate clearance, and the front optic may be reground for any change of power required.

Preformed method

A preformed scleral lens is one whose back surface is a predetermined mathematical form and they may be:

1. Those in which the scleral and optic fittings are done with the same lens.
2. Those which employ separate lenses to assess the scleral and optic fits (Figure 13.8). The latter is the easier method, and a prescription may then be expressed mathematically for the manufacturer, who cuts the lens on a lathe.

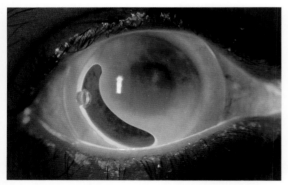

Figure 13.6 Scleral shell with fenestration hole and large limbal bubble. Note that the bubble is tilting the shell to produce heavy touch at the opposite side

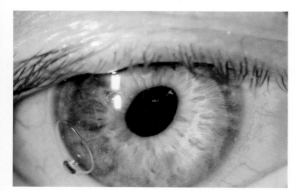

Figure 13.7 Small bubble under a low positioned fenestration hole of a scleral lens

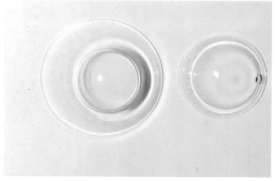

Figure 13.8 Separate lenses to assess the scleral and corneal fits

Scleral lenses are usually marked near the upper periphery, one dot for the right lens and two dots for the left.

Checking a scleral lens

Ask the patient how long they can wear the lenses at a time, and how many periods of wear a day. Any symptoms or problems are noted.

Examination with white light

The limbal bubble must not encroach on the visual axis, and there must be no blanching of conjunctival vessels in the primary eye position, or with any eye movement.

Examination with fluorescein

There should be an adequate corneal clearance, except in keratoconus when there may be some light central corneal touch. The limbal transition zone should be clear, with a circulating air bubble.

Slit-lamp assessment of:

1. Lens edge and surfaces
2. Patency of fenestration hole.
3. Corneal clearance.
4. The cornea for any staining, oedema, infiltrate, scarring or neovascularization.

Insertion and removal of a scleral lens

This is the same whether for the patient or the clinician.

Insertion

Hold lens with finger and thumb and orientate it by the position of the fenestration hole, or channels. With the eye looking down and the upper lids held up with the fingers of the other hand, the lens is placed up under the upper lid. The patient should then look up and the lower lid pulled down so that the lens moves into the correct position under both lids.

Removal

Looking right down, the upper lid is raised and pulled taut so that the upper margin of the scleral lens comes away from the eye. On looking up the lens should be ejected from the eye. Alternatively a suction holder may be placed at the upper margin of the lens to bring the lens down and away from the eye. Patients should be told not to use a finger nail to bring the top of the lens away from the eye, as it can easily result in a corneal abrasion.

Scleral lens to correct ptosis

The scleral lens can be made with a ledge for the upper lid to rest on. Alternatively a horizontal slit may be cut out of the lens above, for the upper lid to rest in (Trodd, 1971). (Figures 13.9 and 13.10.)

Complications of scleral lenses

1. Corneal abrasions may be caused by faulty handling of the lens by the patient.
2. Conjunctival injection and oedema.
3. Corneal oedema, abrasions and bubble impressions.

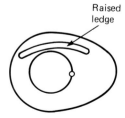

Figure 13.9   Scleral lens with a ptosis ledge

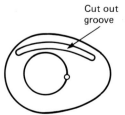

Figure 13.10   Scleral lens with a horizontal slit to correct ptosis

4. Corneal neovascularization, which usually involves all the corneal periphery and requires refitting with rigid corneal lenses (Figure 13.11).

For the future there is a possibility of making scleral lenses from high gas permeable material, to give longer and more comfortable wearing times (Ezekiel, 1983; Pullum, 1987).

Coloured rigid and soft contact lenses

Coloured contact lenses may have either a translucent or opaque tint, or an opaque painted or printed iris area. Reasons for their use include:

Cosmetic

To change or enhance the natural iris colour, which is often requested by actors, actresses, and models.

Prosthetic

To cover corneal opacities and iris defects, and to disguise an unsightly cataract in a blind eye. It may also be used to prevent photophobia, and improve vision in aniridia and albinism.

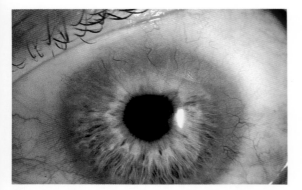

Figure 13.11 Corneal neovascularization in a scleral lens wearer

Tinted rigid lenses

Most rigid lenses are tinted to help the patient to find the lens should it displace from the cornea on to the white of the eye. There is a large range of tints available in PMMA material, but most of the RGP materials are only available in pale blue or pale grey tints, as well as the clear material. The tint should not be too dark, or it will interfere with such activities as night driving. Tinted rigid lenses may be used to disguise unsightly corneal scars, or to enhance a light natural iris colour. A dark brown iris will not be changed in appearance by means of a translucent tint of another colour. To change the colour of the natural iris, the translucent tint needs to be the same colour as the iris and darker, or of an 'additive' colour, i.e. blue iris and yellow tinted lens to produce a green colour. The main problem with rigid lenses is that they do not cover the whole iris, and that they will move with blinking, which can make them obvious to an onlooker. The lenses may be of different tints to distinguish the right and left lenses, particularly for elderly aphakic patients.

Tinted soft lenses

Some soft lens wearers wish to change or enhance their natural iris colour, and this can be done more effectively with a soft than a rigid lens. Most soft lens manufacturers offer a range of tints, which colour the iris only, leaving a clear periphery over the sclera. Many lenses are also available with a clear pupil.

The colour of the tints are variations of blue, green, yellow and brown. A soft lens is more stable on the eye, and will not move excessively. The pupil area may be left clear, or it may be tinted a very dark colour to simulate a black pupil, e.g. to cover a dense white cataract in a blind eye (Figure 13.12). A black occlusive pupil can be used as treatment for amblyopia but needs to be large e.g. 8–10 mm to be really effective. Abadi and Papas (1987) found that in albino patients a high water content dyed pHEMA lens was as effective as shielding the iris as an opaque iris print lens.

Tinted trial lenses are essential for the patient to assess the colour change themselves, before the lenses are ordered, so that the onus for the choice is at least partly on them (Table A8.9 Appendix 8).

In assessing the iris and pupil diameters, it is useful to have soft trial lenses with different iris and pupil diameters. This is more accurate than trying to measure these sizes by other means, and it offers a direct comparison with the other eye, if only one eye is being fitted.

It is now possible to make the iris area of a soft lens opaque and white, and then to tint the opaque area the required colour. This enables the iris colour to be changed, and can even make a brown iris appear blue. This seems an effective method of providing an opaque tint to cover corneal scars, particularly when pigmented, but it may need a lens for both eyes in order to get a reasonable colour match. Opaque tinted lenses are produced by CLM, Igel, Hydron and Coopervision (Table A8.10 in Appendix 8).

A new concept is the Aquarius iris tint 77% water content soft lens by CLM The iris patterns are of three designs: 1. coloured base, 2. radial pattern and 3. corona pattern. The colours are blue, green aqua, and yellow, which may be transparent or opaque (Figure 13.13).

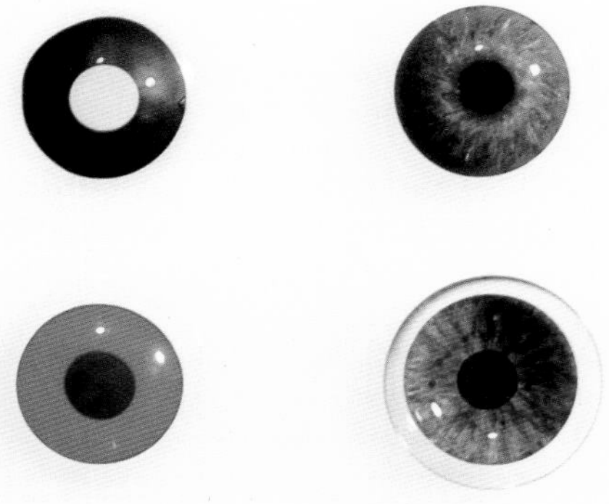

Painted and printed lenses

Rigid corneal lenses may be made with a hand painted laminated iris insert in the lens, to match the iris of the other eye. This will conceal the iris that it covers, and the pupil may be left clear, or be painted black if required to occlude the patient's pupil (Figure 13.12).

A laminated insert may also be put into a soft lens, and either be painted or printed (Figure 13.12). These lenses are made by Ciba Vision in West Germany. They have to be fitted from laminated trial lenses, which makes the fitting more difficult. They are mainly designed to match the colour of the other normal eye. A colour

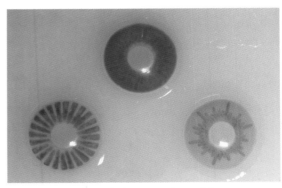

Figure 13.13 'Aquarius' opaque tint soft lenses
Top – coloured base
Left – radial pattern
Right – corona pattern

Figure 13.12 Coloured lenses
Left above – rigid corneal painted lens with clear pupil
Right above – rigid corneal painted lens to hide unsightly blind eye, and to match the other iris
Left below – soft lens with translucent tinted iris, black pupil, and clear scleral area
Right below – laminated painted soft lens for an unsightly blind eye

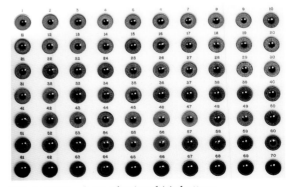

Figure 13.14 A set of painted iris buttons

photograph of the other eye does not give an accurate method of matching. The best method is to have a series of painted iris buttons (Figure 13.14) and to involve the patient in deciding which one is the best match for the other eye. The iris button needs to be held beside the normal eye, and for the patient to compare the two in a mirror, in good natural lighting conditions. The iris button selected is sent to the manufacturer together with the lens specifications, and the iris and pupil diameters required. The pupil may be clear or painted black to occlude the normal pupil. The laminate insert will reduce the oxygen transmissibility, and increase the rigidity of the lens.

Printed iris lenses are available in three colours. When used on one eye only they can occasionally give a reasonable match, but give the best result when fitted to both eyes (Table A8.11 in Appendix 8).

The painted lenses are expensive and take about six months to produce. The results are not always acceptable to the patient, the main problem being the iris and pupil, which are on the front of the cornea. However, despite all the problems, it is often possible to obtain a satisfactory result.

To overcome the delay in obtaining painted soft lenses, Caroline, Harris and Doughman (1980) have suggested a painted iris rigid lens used as part of a piggyback system with a soft lens. The soft lens is lathe cut, and has a disc cut out from its front surface into which the rigid lens fits. For example the overall diameter of the soft lens is 16.00 mm, and its cut out disc is 12 mm diameter. The rigid lens has an overall diameter of 11.80 mm. This piggyback method is also described in Chapter 12.

In the case of a shrunken globe, or lid abnormalities such as ptosis, a cosmetic scleral lens may be required. If this can be a reasonable thickness, it can be possible to make an artificial anterior chamber, which produces a more natural appearance.

References

Scleral lenses

EZEKIEL, D. (1983) Gas permeable haptic lenses. *The Journal of the British Contact Lens Association*, **6**, 158–161

PULLUM, K.W. (1987) Feasibility study for the production of gas permeable scleral lenses using ocular impression techniques. *Transactions of the British Contact Lens Association Annual Clinical Conference No. 4*, 35–39

TRODD, T.C. (1971) Ptosis props in ocular myopathy. *Contact Lens*, **3**, 3–5

Coloured lenses

ABADI, R.V. and PAPAS, E. (1987) Visual performance with artificial iris contact lenses. *The Journal of the British Contact Lens Association*, **10**, 10–15

CAROLINE, P.J., HARRIS, J.K. and DOUGHMAN, M.D. (1980) A new cosmetic piggyback technique for disfigured corneas. *Contact and Intraocular Lens Medical Journal*, **6**, 400–404

Further reading

Scleral lenses

ALLEN, L. and WEBSTER, H.E. (1969) Artificial eye fitting. *American Journal of Ophthalmology*, **67**, 189–217

DALLOS, J. (1937) The individual fitting of contact glasses. *Transactions of the Ophthalmological Society of the UK*, **57**, 509–520

GIRARD, L.J. and SOPER, J.W. (1966) Flush fitting scleral contact lenses. *American Journal of Opthalmology*, **61**, 1109–1122

MARRIOTT, P.J. (1980) Ocular impressions and scleral lens fitting. In *Contact Lenses* (eds J. Stone and A.J. Phillips), 2nd edn, Butterworths, London and Boston, pp. 213–236

WOODWARD, E.G. (1980) Preformed scleral lens fitting techniques. In *Contact Lenses* (eds J. Stone and A.J. Phillips), 2nd edn, Butterworths, London and Boston, pp. 237–255

14

Therapeutic soft contact lenses

Extended wear soft contact lenses may be used in the treatment of certain corneal diseases. Such lenses were commonly called bandage lenses, but the preferred term now is a therapeutic soft contact lens (TSCL). A number of soft lenses are now available for therapeutic use. The main requirement is that they must supply an adequate amount of oxygen to the cornea, and have a large enough OD to be stable on the eye.

The oxygen requirement may be attained in two ways:

1. By increasing the water contant of the lens, as for example the Sauflon PW lens, which has a water content of 79% and a CT 0.18 mm with plano power.
2. By reducing the thickness of a lower water content lens, such as the Syntex CSI EW lens which has a water content of 38.5%, and a CT of only 0.035 mm with plano power.

Examples of some TSCLs and their specifications are given in Table A8.12 in Appendix 8. The thicker higher water content lenses have a larger water reservoir and are especially useful for dry eyes when used with artificial tears (rewetting drops). Thinner lenses are better for protection or to aid healing of the cornea. Basically all TSCLs can be used for the relief of pain due to corneal epithelial defects. By interposing the lens between the cornea and overlying lid, or aberrant lashes, mechanical protection is provided, which will also aid the healing of epithelial defects. TSCLs are usually made with plano power, but may also be powered, as for example when used to treat aphakic bullous keratopathy. The higher water content lenses are more fragile and more prone to develop surface film and deposits. They are also more unreliable optically, due to the greater changes which may occur in their water content when they are being worn. The thinner lower water content lenses vary less in water content and are optically more consistent.

Silicone rubber lenses have been used therapeutically, and the Revlens, a soft acrylic rubber lens is under investigation in the USA.

Fitting a therapeutic lens

A TSCL should only be fitted to a patient who is able and willing to return for follow up examinations, and to follow instructions for treatment.

It is essential that a lens is fitted loose, and not too tight on a cornea with normal epithelium. Failure to do this, particularly on a dry eye, will create a tight fit with lens dehydration, and consequent problems. However, a lens must be fitted with minimum movement on a cornea with a loose epithelium, in order to promote healing. A loose lens will produce friction and rubbing over the corneal surface. Having decided on a suitable water content, a lens of appropriate BOZR and TD is placed on the eye. If keratometry is possible, a lens with a BOZR about 1 mm flatter than the mean K reading is used. A large diameter lens is preferable to increase the lens stability, which helps to reduce lens loss. When the lens has stabilized on the eye, the fit is assessed. If the lens fit is too loose, it may be tightened by reducing the BOZR, or increasing the TD.

Conversely, if the lens fit is too tight, and it does

not have sufficient movement on the eye, the BOZR may be increased, or the TD reduced. It may be necessary to change to a lens from another manufacturer if a suitable one does not exist in the range being used. Most ophthalmologists who use therapeutic lenses, tend to have lenses from two or more manufacturers in stock to cover the two main groups.

Handling

Lenses are stored in sterile N-saline in a sealed container. If a patient has a 'dirty' tear film with much debris, the eye should be irrigated with N-saline drops before inserting the lens. The lens must be put on the eye with as much sterile precaution as possible. The back surface of the lens, which will be in contact with the eye, must never be touched with the fingers. A sterile plastic ointment applicator is useful for removing the lens from its container.

It can often be extremely difficult to insert a lens without trapping some mucus or other debris under it. Should this happen, either massage the upper lid over the lens, or push the lens upwards on the cornea with the lower lid margin, and ask the patient to blink completely closed and open over the lens a few times. This should have the desired effect of expelling any debris from under the lens. If the lens is irritating, and there is still debris under the lens, it should be removed, and its back surface sprayed with unpreserved N-saline from an aerosol can. If debris under the lens is still a problem, put a thicker drop e.g. hypromellose 1% or polyvinyl alcohol (PVA) 1.4%, in the eye before inserting the lens, and any debris still under the lens, should be easier to expel. Holding the lens between the thumb and forefinger at its lower edge gives the best control, and it is less likely to be dropped. The lens can be placed either directly onto the cornea, or under the upper or lower eyelid, whichever is easiest. Tarsorraphies can be a problem when placing the lens on the eye, but can be very useful in preventing lens loss. Removal of a therapeutic soft lens from an eye with damaged epithelium, must be done with great care after previously using copious N-saline drops in the eye, to fully hydrate the lens.

Management

The patient must be taught the importance of correct and adequate blinking, in order to keep the lens well hydrated and clean. This is even more important in the presence of a dry eye. Unpreserved N-saline drops should be used in the mornings, and at any time during the day, depending on the degree of dryness. However, other medication in the form of drops may be required to treat the ocular disease, and these may be helpful in keeping the lens hydrated. If possible unpreserved drops should be used, but when this is not possible those necessary to treat the disease must be used. Patients should be seen the day after having a TSCL put on an eye, and then subsequently at intervals determined by the state of the disease.

Intraocular pressures may be measured over a soft lens either by the McKay–Marg tonometer, or by pneumotonometry (Meyer, Stanifer and Bobb, 1978), without using fluorescein or local anaesthesia.

Indications for therapeutic soft contact lenses

Protection of normal corneal epithelium

Trichiasis

If it is not possible to treat this surgically, a therapeutic lens will prevent the lashes from rubbing the cornea. It is important to use a large diameter lens to prevent a lash getting under the edge of the lens, and for it to be thin with a low water content. Aphakic patients may have some trichiasis, and a TSCL will have the dual function of improving both vision and comfort.

Lid margin deformities

For example entropion, which can be treated with a therapeutic lens as a temporary measure until surgery can be performed.

Protection of corneal graft epithelium

This is important with regard to corneal hydration, and to protect the donor epithelium, and particularly so when the graft has been undertaken for a chemical burn. A high water content TSCL, and frequent applications of artificial tears need to be used. Care must be used to ensure that the corneal graft sutures have not been too deeply placed, as if deep and loose, bacteria can track down the suture into the anterior chamber (Aquavella and Shaw, 1976).

Protection of the epithelium in a dry eye

This requires all methods of improving the tear flow to be used, before trying a therapeutic lens. This includes the frequent applications of artificial tears, preferably preservative free, as well as occlusion of both upper and lower puncta. A TSCL should be kept as a last resort in treatment of a dry eye, because of the risk of infection. The TSCL should have a high water content, and artificial tears or N-saline drops used copiously, to keep the lens and eye well hydrated. If a patient is unable to use artificial tear drops frequently enough, a thinner low water content lens would be preferable. The use of antibiotic drops twice a day as prophylaxis against infection is advisable, if there might be any delay in the patient being seen by an ophthalmologist (Binder and Worthen, 1976).

A TSCL is prone to develop deposits in the dry eye, and will probably need frequent replacement. However, for some patients with extremely dry and painful eyes, the therapeutic lens may be a great help. The patient must be aware of the risks involved, and that they must see an ophthalmologist immediately should problems occur. Dry eyed patients include those with pemphigoid and Stevens Johnson syndrome.

Exposure keratitis from seventh nerve palsy

This may be a temporary condition, and a high water content therapeutic lens can be used together with frequent artificial tears. Inadequate abnormal blinking may cause problems, if the lens becomes dry and tight. A thin lower water content lens may be better. If the condition is permanent a tarsorraphy is preferable.

To aid the healing of abnormal epithelium

Corneal epithelial dystrophies

This includes Cogan's Microcystic epithelial dystrophy, Meesman's dystrophy, Reis–Bucklers dystrophy and map-dot, fingerpoint dystrophy. Recurrent pain is a predominating symptom from epithelial erosions. A thin TSCL should alleviate the pain, and improve the vision.

Chronic corneal ulcers

For example those due to herpes simplex or severe vernal kerato-conjunctivitis with persistent epithelial defects. If the basement membrane is badly damaged, an ulcer may not epithelialize unless protected by a thin TSCL, to allow the basement membrane to reattach first. The lens must be fitted with minimal movement to avoid disturbance to the healing epithelium, but only when there is no longer any evidence of viral replication. Cycloplegics, antibiotic and antiviral drops can be used with the lens in place. If the ulcer has not epithelialized after several weeks, the therapeutic lens should be removed. It can be used for a longer time if thought desirable, but any possible beneficial effect must be offset against the risk of further infection.

Bilateral corneal abrasions

A TSCL can be used on one or both eyes to avoid a pad and bandage (Acheson, Joseph and Spalton, 1987).

Recurrent corneal erosions

If persistent, they can be treated with a TSCL, particularly if pain is a significant problem (Lowe, 1970). Recurrent erosions can be caused by epithelial dysplasia and trauma, and may be associated with diabetes mellitus. If a traumatic abrasion has not healed with a few days a TSCL may aid healing. If the eye is dry a high water content lens should be used, with copious artificial tear drops, or a thin lens if the tear film is adequate, or the patient cannot cope with frequent drops.

Antibiotic drops should be used until the epithelium has healed, and the lens needs to be kept on the eye for a minimum of two or three months, to

ensure that full epithelial reattachment has occurred. Whenever possible, a therapeutic soft lens should be removed at the beginning of a week so that an early recurrence can be seen without delay.

Herpes simplex keratitis

When there is recurrence and persistence of an epithelial defect, but without any indication of viral activity, a thin TSCL may need to be used for several weeks together with cycloplegics, and antibiotics. Herpes zoster keratitis often leads to epithelial breakdown, due to the corneal anaesthesia, and a TSCL should only be used with great care, but can accelerate epithelialization. Antiviral drugs do not help, as they can be toxic to the corneal epithelium.

Chemical, thermal and irradiation burns

These usually produce epithelial defects which persist for many months, and high water content TSCLs may be useful to restore normal corneal epithelialization (Brown, Tragakis and Pearce, 1972). Silicone rubber lenses, can also be used with frequent lubricating drops, and any necessary medical therapy.

Wet filamentary keratitis

This can be treated with thin therapeutic soft lenses for rapid relief of the discomfort caused by the corneal filaments (Bloomfield *et al.*, 1973). The filaments should be gently removed from the cornea, before applying the lens. If the eye is dry there is a marked risk of infection and it is safer not to use a TSCL. If a TSCL is used, copious artificial tears and acetyl cysteine drops are required.

Neurotrophic keratitis

This has been treated successfully by a TSCL, but the anaesthetic eye is highly susceptible to infection, particularly if it is dry. As for exposure keratitis, a tarsorrhaphy is the preferred treatment.

Thygeson's superficial punctate keratitis

This responds well to topical steroids, but they may need to be used for lengthy periods because of recurrences. Alternatively thin therapeutic soft lenses can provide symptomatic relief, and rapid healing of the lesions. However, the lesions may recur soon after removal of the lenses (Goldberg, Schanzlin and Brown, 1980).

Moulding and splinting

Following keratoplasty

When lifting or displacement of the graft occurs, a thin therapeutic soft lens can be used, to help flatten and reposition the graft (Aquavella and Shaw, 1976). It can also be useful if 'cheese-wiring' of the corneal graft sutures occurs. The main risk of using a TSCL is infection, and precautions should be taken by using the lens for as short a time as possible, and with antibiotic drops.

Deep corneal ulcers and Descemetoceles

If these are liable to perforate they can be treated with a temporary TSCL

Wound leaks

These can be plugged by a TSCL, and a small corneal perforation needs a tight fitting TSCL, so that any secondary stromal swelling will help to seal the perforation. Tissue adhesives such as isobutyl cyano acrylate, can be used to fix the lens on the cornea.

Relief of pain

Bullous keratopathy

This occurs as a result of endothelial failure, so that the cornea becomes oedematous. Initially it is mainly stromal oedema which produces a deterioration of vision, which is typically worse on awakening. During the day, due to surface evaporation vision may clear. In more advanced bullous keratopathy, bullae may arise on the surface, and rupture causing pain. A thin TSCL can prevent bullae forming and so relieve the pain. It should improve the vision, so long as there are not too many folds in Descemets membrane. A TSCL can be worn continuously for many years if required for the treatment for bullous keratopathy, which is the indication par excellence for a TSCL (Liebowitz and Rosenthal, 1971).

Drug delivery

Therapeutic soft lenses have been used to obtain a higher concentration of a drug in contact with the eye for a longer time. The dehydrated lens is soaked in a solution of the drug, and worn on the eye for the required length of time. Drugs which have been used in this way are pilocarpine, antibiotics, steroids, and the antivirals.

An 'Ocusert' is a reservoir of pilocarpine between two membranes, which is worn in the upper or lower fornix. As it is expensive and often uncomfortable, it has not gained popularity in the UK.

Therapeutic soft lens complications

When using a TSCL the complications which may occur from using the lens, must be borne in mind, and also that one is dealing with compromised defences. An attempt must be made to differentiate between a true complication, and a therapeutic failure, which is not always easy. The complications include:

1. Tight lenses which should be changed for a looser fit, or a smaller diameter lens. If the lens is too loose, change for a tighter fit or a larger diameter.
2. Displacement, loss, and damage to the lens is often due to rubbing the eye inadvertently, particularly when sleeping.
3. Lens surface film and deposits, particularly with dry eyes, which are less likely to occur when eye drops are used frequently. Some patients may need frequent lens replacements for this problem.
4. Corneal oedema, may be acute or chronic. Acute corneal oedema may occur if a lens is fitted too tightly or has too low an oxygen transmissability. In severe cases the soft lens must be removed, and a more suitable lens used when the oedema has fully subsided. Should acute corneal oedema recur, the therapeutic soft lens should be discontinued. A mild chronic corneal oedema could be progressive, and may lead to corneal vascularization.
5. Corneal vascularization is normally undesirable, and usually superficial; it should regress on removal of the lens. The causative factors are probably hypoxia and trauma. It may have to be accepted if the lens is otherwise producing the required result, and if the vascularization is not encroaching on the visual axis. In the treatment of chemical burns, and stromal ulceration, corneal vascularization will aid healing and is desirable. Vascularization usually originates at the upper limbus, but may also originate at the limbus nearest to the area of stromal pathology. Deep vascularization may occur if hypoxia and trauma are more severe.
6. Sterile corneal infiltrates are usually asymptomatic and peripheral, and usually clear with lens removal, without treatment. It is safer to treat them as infective corneal ulcers with appropriate investigations and treatment.
7. Sterile hypopyon occurring without a corneal infiltrate, should resolve by removing the soft lens, and using mydriatics. If the hypopyon occurs in the presence of a corneal infiltrate, infection is a possibility, and full diagnostic and therapeutic measures should be done. Bacterial ulcers may occur with therapeutic soft lenses, as the eye being treated is likely to be prone to infection, particularly if dry. Prophylactic antibiotic drops can be used, but are often ineffective. As *Pseudomonas* is a common infecting organism, full diagnostic and therapeutic measures must be instituted as rapidly as possible (Brown *et al.*, 1974).

Any patient wearing a TSCL should have explicit instructions about their medication, and should be told to see an ophthalmologist immediately should they have any pain, discharge, blurring of vision, or any increased redness of the eye wearing the lens.

References

ACHESON, J.F., JOSEPH, J. and SPALTON, D.J. (1987) Use of contact lenses in an eye casualty department for the primary treatment of traumatic corneal abrasions. *British Journal of Ophthalmology*, **71**, 285–289

AQUAVELLA, J.V. and SHAW, E.L. (1976) Hydrophilic bandages in penetrating keratoplasty. *Annals of Ophthalmology*, **8**, 1207–1219

BINDER, P.S. and WORTHEN, D.M. (1976) A continuous wear hydrophilic lens: Prophylactic topical antibiotics. *Archives of Ophthalmology*, **94**, 2109–2111

BLOOMFIELD, S.E., GASSET, A.R., FORSTER, S.L and BROWN, S.I. (1973) Treatment of filamentary keratitis with the soft contact lens. *American Journal of Ophthalmology*, **76**, 978–980

BROWN, S.I., TRAGAKIS, M.P. and PEARCE, D.B. (1972) Treatment of the alkali burned cornea. *American Journal of Ophthalmology*, **74**, 316–320

BROWN, S.I., BLOOMFIELD, S., PEARCE, D.B. and TRAGAKIS, M. (1974) Infections with the therapeutic soft lens. *Archives of Ophthalmology*, **91**, 275–277

GOLDBERG, D.B., SCHANZLIN, D.J. and BROWN, S.I. (1980) Management of Thygeson's superficial punctate keratitis. *American Journal of Ophthalmology*, **89**, 22–24

LIEBOWITZ, H.M. and ROSENTHAL, P.R. (1971) Hydrophilic contact lenses in the treatment of bullous keratopathy. *American Journal of Ophthalmology*, **85**, 162

LOWE, R.F. (1970) Recurrent erosion of the cornea. *British Journal of Ophthalmology*, **54**, 805–809

MEYER, R.F., STANIFER, R.M. and BOBB, K.C. (1978) McKay-Marg tonometry over therapeutic soft contact lenses. *American Journal of Ophthalmology*, **86**, 19

Further reading

BALDONE, J.A. and KAUFMAN, H.E. (1983) Soft contact lenses and clinical disease. *American Journal of Ophthalmology*, **95**, 851–852

DOHLMAN, C.H., BARUCHOFF, S.A. and MOBILIA, E. (1973) Complications in use of soft contact lenses in corneal disease. *Archives of Ophthalmology*, **90**, 367–371

GASSET, A.R. and KAUFMAN, H.E. (1970) Therapeutic uses of hydrophilic contact lenses. *American Journal of Ophthalmology*, **69**, 252–259

KHTDADOUST, A.A., SILVERSTEIN, A.M., KENYON, K.R. and DOWLING, J.E. (1969) Adhesion of regenerating corneal epithelium: The role of basement membrane. *American Journal of Ophthalmology*, **65**, 339–348

Appendix 1

Comparative methods of recording visual acuity

UK	USA	VISUS
6/60	20/200	0.10
6/36	20/120	0.16
6/24	20/80	0.25
6/18	20/60	0.30
6/12	20/40	0.50
6/9	20/30	0.65
6/6	20/20	1.00
6/5	20/15	

Appendix 2

Centre thickness chart for PMMA lenses

Power (DS)	Centre thickness	Power (DS)	Centre thickness
−12.0 and over	0.08	Reduced Front Optics	
−11.00	0.09	+ 6.00	0.26
−10.00	0.10	+ 7.00	0.27
− 9.00	0.11	+ 8.00	0.28
− 8.00	0.12	+ 9.00	0.29
− 7.00	0.13	+10.00	0.30
− 6.00	0.14	+11.00	0.32
− 5.00	0.15	+12.00	0.33
− 4.00	0.17	+13.00	0.35
− 3.00	0.19	+14.00	0.36
− 2.00	0.21	+15.00	0.37
− 1.00	0.22	+16.00	0.39
PLANO	0.24	+17.00	0.40
+ 1.00	0.25	+18.00	0.42
+ 2.00	0.27	+19.00	0.43
+ 3.00	0.28	+20.00	0.45
+ 4.00	0.30		
+ 5.00	0.34		

Courtesy of Global Contact Lenses

Appendix 3

Radius of curvature to dioptric power chart for refractive index of 1.3375

Radius	Dioptres	Radius	Dioptres	Radius	Dioptres
9.00	37.50	8.00	42.19	7.00	48.21
8.95	37.71	7.95	42.45	6.90	48.91
8.90	37.72	7.90	42.72	6.80	49.63
8.85	38.14	7.85	42.99	6.70	50.37
8.80	38.35	7.80	43.27	6.60	51.14
8.75	38.57	7.75	43.55	6.50	51.92
8.70	38.79	7.70	43.83	6.40	52.73
8.65	39.02	7.65	44.19	6.30	53.57
8.60	39.24	7.60	44.41	6.20	54.43
8.55	39.47	7.55	44.70	6.10	55.33
8.50	39.71	7.50	45.00	6.00	56.25
8.45	39.94	7.45	45.30	5.90	57.20
8.40	40.18	7.40	45.61	5.80	58.19
8.35	40.42	7.35	45.92	5.70	59.21
8.30	40.66	7.30	46.23	5.60	60.29
8.25	40.91	7.25	45.55	5.50	61.36
8.20	41.16	7.20	46.87	5.40	62.50
8.15	41.41	7.15	47.20	5.30	63.68
8.10	41.67	7.10	47.53	5.20	64.90
8.05	41.92	7.05	47.87	5.10	66.18

Adapted from *Contact Lenses* by Stone and Phillips (second edition) Butterworths

Appendix 4

Effective power of contact lenses allowing for the back vertex distance of a spectacle lens

Spectacle refraction	Vertex distance 8mm	10mm	12mm	14mm	16mm
− 2.50D	− 2.45D	− 2.44D	− 2.43D	− 2.42 D	− 2.40D
− 3.00	2.93	2.91	2.90	2.88	2.86
− 3.50	3.40	3.38	3.36	3.34	3.31
− 4.00	3.88	3.85	3.82	3.79	3.76
− 4.50	4.34	4.31	4.27	4.23	4.20
− 5.00	4.81	4.76	4.72	4.67	4.63
− 5.50	5.27	5.21	5.16	5.11	5.06
− 6.00	5.72	5.66	5.60	5.53	5.47
− 6.50	6.18	6.11	6.03	5.96	5.89
− 7.00	6.63	6.54	6.46	6.38	6.30
− 7.50	7.08	6.98	6.88	6.79	6.70
− 8.00	7.52	7.41	7.30	7.19	7.09
− 8.50	7.96	7.84	7.72	7.60	7.49
− 9.00	8.40	8.26	8.12	7.99	7.87
− 9.50	8.83	8.67	8.53	8.38	8.24
−10.00	9.26	9.09	8.93	8.77	8.62
−10.50	9.69	9.50	9.32	9.15	8.99
−11.00	10.11	9.91	9.72	9.53	9.35
−11.50	10.53	10.31	10.11	9.90	9.71
−12.00	10.95	10.71	10.49	10.27	10.07
−12.50	11.36	11.11	10.87	10.64	10.42
−13.00	11.78	11.50	11.25	11.00	10.76
−13.50	12.18	11.89	11.62	11.35	11.10
−14.00	12.59	12.28	11.99	11.71	11.44
−14.50	12.99	12.66	12.35	12.05	11.77
−15.00	13.39	13.04	12.71	12.40	12.10
−15.50	13.79	13.42	13.07	12.74	12.42
−16.00	14.18	13.79	13.42	13.07	12.74
−16.50	14.57	14.16	13.77	13.40	13.05
−17.00	14.96	14.53	14.12	13.73	13.36
−17.50	15.35	14.89	14.46	14.06	13.67
−18.00	15.74	15.25	14.80	14.38	13.98
−18.50	16.12	15.61	15.14	14.70	14.28
−19.00	16.49	15.97	15.47	15.01	14.57
−19.50	16.87	16.32	15.80	15.32	14.86
−20.00	17.24	16.67	16.13	15.63	15.15

Spectacle refraction	Vertex distance 8mm	10mm	12mm	14mm	16mm
+ 2.50D	+2.55D	+2.56D	+2.58D	+2.59D	+2.60D
+ 3.00	3.07	3.09	3.11	3.13	3.15
+ 3.50	3.60	3.63	3.65	3.68	3.71
+ 4.00	4.13	4.17	4.20	4.24	4.27
+ 4.50	4.67	4.71	4.76	4.80	4.85
+ 5.00	5.21	5.26	5.32	5.38	5.43
+ 5.50	5.75	5.82	5.89	5.96	6.03
+ 6.00	6.30	6.38	6.47	6.55	6.64
+ 6.50	6.86	6.95	7.05	7.15	7.26
+ 7.00	7.42	7.53	7.64	7.76	7.88
+ 7.50	7.98	8.11	8.24	8.38	8.52
+ 8.00	8.55	8.70	8.85	9.01	9.17
+ 8.50	9.12	9.29	9.47	9.65	9.84
+ 9.00	9.70	9.89	10.09	10.30	10.51
+ 9.50	10.28	10.49	10.72	10.95	11.20
+10.00	10.87	11.11	11.36	11.63	11.90
+10.50	11.46	11.73	12.01	12.31	12.62
+11.00	12.06	12.36	12.67	13.00	13.35
+11.50	12.66	12.99	13.34	13.71	14.09
+12.00	13.27	13.64	14.02	14.42	14.85
+12.50	13.89	14.29	14.71	15.15	15.63
+13.00	14.51	14.94	15.40	15.89	16.41
+13.50	15.14	15.61	16.11	16.65	17.22
+14.00	15.77	16.28	16.83	17.41	18.04
+14.50	16.40	16.96	17.56	18.20	18.88
+15.00	17.04	17.65	18.29	18.99	19.74
+15.50	17.69	18.34	19.04	19.79	20.61
+16.00	18.35	19.05	19.80	20.62	21.51
+16.50	19.01	19.76	20.57	21.45	22.42
+17.00	19.68	20.48	21.36	22.31	23.35
+17.50	20.35	21.21	22.15	23.18	24.31
+18.00	21.03	21.95	22.96	24.06	25.28

Appendix 5

Alterations to contact lens power when changing to a steeper or flatter fit

Corneal radius (mm)	Back optic radius of lens fitted steeper than corneal radius by							
	0.05mm	0.10mm	0.15mm	0.20mm	0.25mm	0.30mm	0.35mm	0.40mm
6.5	−0.40D	−0.81D	−1.22D	−1.64D	−2.07D	−2.50D	−2.94D	−3.39D
6.6	0.39	0.78	1.18	1.59	2.00	2.42	2.85	3.29
6.7	0.38	0.76	1.15	1.54	1.94	2.35	2.76	3.18
6.8	0.37	0.74	1.12	1.50	1.89	2.28	2.68	3.09
6.9	0.35	0.71	1.08	1.45	1.83	2.21	2.60	2.99
7.0	0.35	0.70	1.05	1.41	1.78	2.15	2.53	2.91
7.1	0.34	0.68	1.03	1.38	1.73	2.09	2.46	2.83
7.2	0.32	0.65	0.99	1.33	1.68	2.03	2.38	2.74
7.3	0.32	0.64	0.96	1.29	1.63	1.97	2.32	2.67
7.4	0.31	0.62	0.94	1.26	1.58	1.91	2.25	2.59
7.5	0.30	0.61	0.92	1.23	1.55	1.87	2.19	2.52
7.6	0.29	0.59	0.89	1.20	1.51	1.82	2.14	2.46
7.7	0.28	0.57	0.86	1.16	1.46	1.77	2.08	2.39
7.8	0.28	0.56	0.84	1.13	1.42	1.72	2.02	2.33
7.9	0.27	0.55	0.83	1.11	1.39	1.68	1.97	2.27
8.0	0.26	0.53	0.80	1.08	1.35	1.64	1.92	2.21
8.1	0.26	0.52	0.78	1.05	1.32	1.60	1.83	2.16
8.2	0.25	0.50	0.76	1.02	1.28	1.55	1.82	2.10
8.3	0.25	0.50	0.75	1.00	1.26	1.52	1.78	2.05
8.4	0.24	0.48	0.73	0.98	1.23	1.48	1.74	2.00
8.5	0.23	0.47	0.71	0.95	1.20	1.45	1.70	1.95

Corneal radius (mm)	Back optic radius of lens fitted flatter than corneal radius by					
	0.05mm	0.10mm	0.15mm	0.20mm	0.25mm	0.30mm
6.5	+0.39D	+0.78D	+1.16D	+1.54D	+1.91D	+2.28D
6.6	0.39	0.76	1.13	1.50	1.86	2.21
6.7	0.37	0.74	1.10	1.45	1.80	2.15
6.8	0.36	0.71	1.06	1.41	1.75	2.09
6.9	0.35	0.70	1.04	1.38	1.71	2.03
7.0	0.34	0.68	1.01	1.33	1.65	1.97
7.1	0.33	0.65	0.97	1.29	1.60	1.91
7.2	0.32	0.64	0.95	1.26	1.57	1.87
7.3	0.31	0.62	0.93	1.23	1.53	1.82
7.4	0.31	0.61	0.91	1.20	1.49	1.77
7.5	0.30	0.59	0.88	1.16	1.44	1.72
7.6	0.29	0.57	0.85	1.13	1.41	1.68
7.7	0.28	0.56	0.84	1.11	1.38	1.64
7.8	0.28	0.55	0.82	1.08	1.34	1.60
7.9	0.27	0.53	0.79	1.05	1.30	1.55
8.0	0.26	0.52	0.77	1.02	1.27	1.52
8.1	0.25	0.50	0.75	1.00	1.24	1.48
8.2	0.25	0.50	0.74	0.98	1.22	1.45
8.3	0.24	0.48	0.72	0.96	1.18	1.41
8.4	0.24	0.47	0.70	0.93	1.16	1.38
8.5	0.23	0.46	0.69	0.91	1.13	1.35

Reprinted by kind permission of the Association of British Dispensing Opticians

Appendix 6

Oxygen transmissibility conversion table

t \ *Dk*	5	10	15	20	30	40	50	60	70	80	90
0.05	10.0	20.0	30.0	40.0	60.0	80.0	100.0	120.0	140.0	160.0	180.0
0.06	8.3	16.6	25.0	33.3	50.0	66.6	83.3	100.0	116.6	133.3	150.0
0.07	7.1	14.3	21.4	28.5	42.8	57.1	71.4	85.7	100.0	114.2	128.5
0.08	6.3	12.5	18.8	25.0	37.5	50.0	62.5	75.0	87.5	100.0	112.5
0.09	5.5	11.1	16.7	22.2	33.3	44.4	55.5	66.6	77.7	88.8	100.0
0.10	5.0	10.0	15.0	20.0	30.0	40.0	50.0	60.0	70.0	80.0	90.0
0.11	4.5	9.1	13.6	18.1	27.2	36.3	45.4	54.5	63.6	72.7	81.8
0.12	4.1	8.3	12.5	16.6	25.0	33.0	41.6	50.0	58.3	66.6	75.0
0.13	3.8	7.7	11.5	15.4	23.0	30.7	38.4	46.1	53.8	61.5	69.2
0.14	3.6	7.1	10.7	14.3	21.4	28.5	35.7	42.8	50.0	57.1	64.2
0.15	3.3	6.6	10.0	13.3	23.0	26.6	33.3	40.0	46.6	53.3	60.0
0.16	3.1	6.3	9.4	12.5	18.7	25.0	31.2	37.5	43.7	50.0	56.2
0.17	2.9	5.9	8.8	11.7	17.6	23.5	29.4	35.2	41.1	47.0	52.9
0.18	2.8	5.6	8.3	11.1	16.6	22.2	27.7	33.3	38.8	44.4	50.0
0.19	2.6	5.3	7.9	10.5	15.7	21.0	26.3	31.5	36.8	42.1	47.3
0.20	2.5	5.0	7.5	10.0	15.0	20.0	25.0	30.0	35.0	40.0	45.0
0.30	1.6	3.3	5.0	6.6	10.0	13.3	16.6	20.0	23.3	26.6	30.0
0.40	1.2	2.5	3.7	5.0	7.5	10.0	12.5	15.0	17.5	20.0	22.5

Dk = gas permeability of lens material
t = geometric centre thickness of the lens

Appendix 7

Preparations for use with contact lenses

Hard contact lenses

Abatron

Amiclean solution (C) THM 0.01 and CHX 0.005, Ami-10 (S/D) THM 0.001 and CHX 0.005

Alcon

Clens (C) BKC 0.02, Pliagel (C) sorbic acid 0.1, Soaclens (S/D) BKC 0.01, Adapettes (RW) THM 0.002

Allergan

Clean-n-Soak (C and S/D) PMN 0.004, LC65 (C) THM 0.001 EDTA, Total (S/D and W) BKC 0.004 PVA 2.5, Liquifilm Wetting (W) BKC 0.004 PVA 2.0.

Barnes Hind

Cleaning and Soaking (C) BKC 0.01, Titan (C) BKC 0.02, Intensive Cleaner (C) THM 0.001, Soquette (S/D) BKC 0.01, Wetting and Soaking (S/D) BKC 0.005, Wetting (W) BKC 0.004, Comfort Drops (RW) BKC 0.005, One Solution (C, W, S/D) BKC 0.01

Boots

Cleaning, Soaking and Wetting CHX 0.06 BKC 0.004 EDTA 0.128

132

Ciba Vision Contactasol

Contactaclean (C) Contactasoak (S/D) and Contactasol (W) all contain BKC 0.004, CHX 0.006 EDTA 0.128. 02 Care* (C) BKC 0.005 EDTA 0.12 TE Cleaning (C) THM 0.0025 and CHX 0.0025, TE Storage and Rinsing (S/D and W) THM 0.0025 and CHX 0.0025

Coopervision

Kelsoak (2) (C and S/D) and Kelvinol (2) (W) BKC 0.004 CHX 0.006 EDTA 0.128

Polymer Technology

The Boston Lens Cleaner (C), Boston Lens Wetting and Soaking Solution (S/D and W) CHX 0.006 EDTA 0.6

Sauflon Pharmaceuticals

Stericlens (C and W) THM 0.004 EDTA 0.1, Sterisoak (S/D) BKC 0.002 CHB 0.4 EDTA 0.1

Smith and Nephew

Transol (W), Transoak BKC 0.01 EDTA 0.2, Transdrop (RW) BKC 0.004

Key to use of preparations (C) Cleaning, (S/D) Soaking and Disinfecting, (W) Wetting, (RW) Rewetting

*Specifically for use with Menicon O2 gas permeable lenses.

Key to antimicrobials BKC – benzalkonium chloride; CHX – chlorhexidine digluconate; THM – thiomersal (thimerosal); PVA – polyvinyl alcohol; CHB – chlorbutol; PMN – phenylmercuric nitrate; EDTA – sodium edetate

Soft contact lenses

Abatron

Amiclean solution (DC) THM 0.001 CHX 0.005, Ami-10 (S/D) THM 0.001 CHX 0.005; Amidose Saline (R) NA, Amiclair Enzyme Tabs (protease, lipase and pronase)

Alcon

Preflex (DC) THM 0.004, Pliagel (DC) sorbic acid 0.1, Flexcare and Flexsol (S/D), Normol (R) THM 0.001, CHX 0.005, Adapettes (RW) THM 0.002, Sterilettes (RW) THM 0.002, Softab Tabs (S/D) chlorine (DIC), Salettes (B and R) NA, Spray Saline (B and R) NA

Allergan Hydrocare

Cleaning and Soaking (DC and S/D) THM 0.001 QUAT 0.013, LC 65 (DC) THM 0.001 EDTA, Boiling/Rinsing (B and R), Preserved Saline (B and R) THM 0.002 EDTA 0.01, Liquifilm Tears (RW) CHB 0.5, Hydrocare Fizzy Protein Removing Tablets (papain), Lens Plus unpreserved saline, Oxysept 1 3% H_2O_2, Oxysept 2 Catalase

Barnes Hind

Cleaner No.4 (DC) THM 0.001, Intensive Cleaner Solution (C) THM 0.001 Hexidin (S/D) THM 0.002 CHX 0.003, Soft Therm (B and R) THM 0.001, Soft Comfort (RW) THM 0.004, Softmate Protein Removing Solution NA

Bausch and Lomb

Daily Cleaner (DC) sorbic acid, B and L Soaking (S/D) THM 0.002 QUAT 0.03, Lens Lubricant (RW) THM 0.004, Saline solution (B and R) THM 0.001, Saline Aerosol NA, SB1 Saline (R) sorbic acid, B and L Fizzy Protein Tabs (papain)

Boots

Daily Cleaner Soaking (S/D) and Comfort Drops (RW) THM 0.0025 CHX 0.0025 EDTA

Ciba Vision Contactasol

Hydroclean (DC), Hydrosoak (S/D) and Hydrosol (RW) THM 0.0025 CHX 0.0025 EDTA 0.128 10/10 H_2O_2 3%, 10/10 Neutraliser (R) 0.5 pyruvate and N-saline, Solar Saline Aerosol NA
TE Cleaning (C) THM 0.0025 CHX 0.0025, TE Storage and Rinsing THM 0.0025 CHX 0.0025, Lensept (C) H_2O_2 3%, Lensrins (and catalyst) (R) THM 0.001 EDTA 0.1, Miraflow (DC) IPA, Mirasoak (S/D) THM 0.001 CHX 0.005 EDTA 0.1, Clerz (RW) Unit dose NA

Coopervision

Mediclean (DC) and Medisoak (S/D) THM 0.0025 CHX 0.0025 EDTA 0.128

Hydron

Cleaning (DC) and Soaking (S/D) CHX 0.002, Comfort (RW) THM 0.002 CHX 0.001 EDTA 0.1, Solusal Saline Aerosol NA, Saline B Na phosphate 0.227 Na acid phosphate 0.062

ICN

Unicare (DC and S/D) THM 0.0015, Eyefresh (C and R) THM 0.001

Sauflon Pharmaceuticals

Sterisolv (DC) THM 0.004 EDTA 0.1, Sterisal 2 (S/D) THM 0.002 CHX 0.002 EDTA 0.1, Aerosol Saline NA, Aerotabs tablets (S/D) Chlorine (Halazone)

Smith and Nephew

Prymeclean (C) CHX 0.002, Prymesoak (S/D) CHX 0.002

Key to function of preparations (B) Boiling, (R) Rinsing, (S/D) Soaking and Disinfecting, (DC) Daily Cleaner, (RW) Rewetting

Key to antimicrobial present CHB – chlorbutol; DIC – dichloroisocynaurate; IPA – isopropyl alcohol; QUAT – quaternary ammonium base; NA – no antimicrobial present; CHX – chlorhexidine digluconate; EDTA – sodium edetate; PMN – phenylmercuric nitrate; THM – thiomersal (thimerosal)

Appendix 8

Examples of different types of contact lens

Table A8.1 Examples of available rigid gas permeable lenses

Manufacturer/ Lens	Material	Manufacture	Wetting angle	Dk at 35°C	Diameter (mm)	BOZR (mm)	Powers in dioptres
Bausch and Lomb							
OPL	Amefocon	SC	14.1	14	9.2	7.30 to 8.25 in 0.05 steps	−0.25 to −6.0 in 0.25 steps
HGP	Itafocon A	LC	20	14.6	9.2	As for OPL	+4.0 to −5.0 in 0.25 steps, +4.0 to +6.0 and −5.0 to −12.0 in 0.5 steps
Ciba Vision							
Persecon CE	Sil/PMMA	LC	22	54	8.8	7.2 to 8.4	
					9.3	7.3 to 8.5	+25.0 to −25.0 in 0.25
					9.8	7.3 to 8.5	steps
					10.3	7.4 to 8.6	
Persecon E	CAB	LC	22	8	As for PCE	As for PCE	As for PCE
Contact Lenses Manufacturing							
Metro GP 32	Fluoro MA Siloxanyl-MA	LC	20	32	9.6	7.4 to 8.4 in 0.5 steps	+10.0 to −10.0 in 0.25 steps, +10.5 to +20.0 and −10.50 to −2.00 in 0.50 steps
Metro GP 52	As for 32	LC		52	9.6	As for 32	As for 32
Hydron							
GP 20	Sil/Acr	LC	24	18	9.2, 9.7	7.5 to 8.2 in 0.05 steps	+20.0 to −20.0 up to +10.0 in 0.25 steps then 0.5 steps
GP 50	Sil/Acr	LC	26	54			
Nissel							
Excel 02			complete	16.7	All	All	All
Pilkington/Syntex							
Polycon II	Sil/Acr	LC	15	12	8.5	7.1 to 8.35	Plano to −8.0
					9.0	7.2 to 8.45	+6.0 to −8.0
					9.5	7.2 to 8.65	+6.0 to −10.0
					10.0		+8.25 to +20.0
Polycon HDK	Sil/Acr	LC	25	50	9.0, 9.5	7.0 to 8.6 in 0.05 steps	+15.0 to −15.0 in 0.25 steps

Manufacturer/ Lens	Material	Manufacture	Wetting angle	Dk at 35°C	Diameter (mm)	BOZR (mm)	Powers in dioptres
Optacryl Inc							
Optacryl Z	Polyacrylate/Sil	LC	30	84	All	All	All
Optacryl 2	Sil/Acr	LC	20	84	All	All	All
Paragon Optical Inc							
Paraperm O$_2$	Sil/Acr	LC	23	15.6	All	All	All
Paraperm EW	Sil/Acr	LC	26	56	All	All	All
Paraperm O$_2$+	Sil/Acr	LC	25	39	All	All	All
Polymer Technology							
Boston II		LC	20	14.6	All	All	All
Boston IV		LC	17	26.3	All	All	All
Equalens	Sil/Acr	LC	30	71	All	All	All
Quantum	Fluo/Sil	LC		92	9.6, 10.2	7.2 to 8.4 in 0.50 steps	+4.0 to −7.0 in 0.25 steps, +4.5 to +9.0 and −7.5 to −15.0 in 0.5 steps
Visual Eyes (Ophthalmics)							
Menicon SP		LC	20	32	9.6	7.4 to 8.4 in 0.05 steps	−1.0 to −8.0 in 0.25 steps
Menicon EX				52	9.6	As for MSP	As for MSP
Wohlk							
Hartflex	CAB	Moulded		4.2	8.5, 9.0, 9.5, 10.0, 10.50	6.0 to 8.8 in 0.50 steps	+28.0 to −28.0 in 0.25 steps
Conflex	CAB/EVA	Moulded		7.69 at 21°C	9.4 to 10.4 in 0.5 steps	7.25 to 8.75 in 0.05 steps	+20.0 to −20.0 in 0.25 steps
Silflex	Silicone rubber	Moulded		79.8	11.2, 11.7, 12.7, 13.2	7.3 to 9.0 in 0.25 steps	+20.0 to −20.0 in 0.25 steps (all lenses lenticular)

Table A8.2 Examples of available daily wear soft contact lenses

Manufacturer/ Lens	Water %	BOZR (mm)	Diameter (mm)	CT at −3.00 DS	Powers (DS)	Wearing time	Material and remarks
UNITED KINGDOM							
Bausch and Lomb							
Optima 38	38	Flat and steep	14.0	0.06			pHEMA spuncast and lathed
Ciba Vision							
Weicon 38E	38	Flat and steep	13.0, 13.8, 14.6	0.08	+20.0 to −20.0 (above +10.0 in 0.50 steps)	DW	pHEMA elliptical back curve
Weicon CE	60	Flat and steep	13.0, 13.8, 14.6	0.09	+25.0 to −25.0	DW and EW	Non pHEMA elliptical back curve
Ciba soft Visitint	38	8.3, 8.6, 8.9	13.8	0.07	+6.0 to −8.0 (from above −6.0 in 0.50 steps)	DW	pHEMA with 5% blue tint, moulded spherical back surface

Manufacturer/ Lens	Water %	BOZR (mm)	Diameter (mm)	CT at −3.00 DS	Powers (DS)	Wearing time	Material and remarks
Contact Lenses Manufacturing							
Sauflon 70%	70	7.8, 8.0, 8.2, 8.4, 8.6, 8.8, 9.0	13.0, 13.7, 14.4	0.20	+10.0 to −10.0 in 0.25 steps, −10.5 to −20.0 and +10.5 to +20.0 in 0.50 steps	DW	Non pHEMA
Sauflon 77%	77	7.5, 7.8, 8.1, 8.4, 8.7	13.0, 13.7, 14.4	0.18	+10.0 to −10.0 in 0.25 steps, +10.5 to +20.0 and −10.5 to −20.0 in 0.50 steps	DW and EW	Non pHEMA
Coopervision							
Cooperthin	38	8.4 8.6	14.0 14.5	0.07	Plano to −10.0, −5.0 to −10.0 in 0.50 steps	DW	pHEMA cast moulded
Eurothin	38	8.3, 8.6	13.8	0.07	+8.0 to −10.0	DW	pHEMA lathe cut
Eurolens	38	7.8 to 8.8 in 0.2 steps	13.0	0.12	+8.0 to −8.0	DW	pHEMA lathe cut
Hydron Europe							
Zero 6	38	8.4, 8.7	14.00		Plano to −20.0	DW	
Zero F	38	9.0, 9.3			Plano to +20.0		
Mini	38	7.9 to 8.9 8.1 to 9.3 in 0.2 steps	12.5 13.0	0.12	+30.0 to −30.0	DW	
Zero 4	38	8.3	13.8	0.04	Plano to −7.5	DW or EW	
Spincast	38	8.5 for −3.0 DS	13.5, 14.5	0.07	Plano to −8.0	DW	Cast moulded
Pilkington Barnes Hind							
Softmate I	45	8.7 9.0	14.3 14.8	0.05	Plano to −6.0 in 0.25 steps	DW and EW	Non pHEMA
Softmate II	55	8.7 9.0 9.0	14.3 14.3 14.8	0.05	+7.0 to −12.0 in 0.25 steps	DW and EW	Non pHEMA
Hydrocurve II 45	45	8.3, 8.6 8.9	13.5 14.5	0.05	+20.0 to −20.0 in 0.25 steps	DW and EW	Non pHEMA
Hydrocurve II 55	55	8.5 8.8	14.0 14.5	0.05	+20.0 to −12.0 in 0.25 steps	DW and EW	Non pHEMA
Custom Eyes	45	8.7 9.0	14.3 14.8	0.07	+7.0 to −12.0 in 0.25 steps	DW	Non pHEMA
Softmate B							
Elite	55	8.8	14.5		Plano to −6.0 in 0.25 steps		Treated non pHEMA

Manufacturer/ Lens	Water %	BOZR (mm)	Diameter (mm)	CT at −3.00 DS	Powers (DS)	Wearing time	Material and remarks
Pilkington Contact Lenses							
CS1	38.5	8.3, 8.6, 8.9, 9.2	13.8	0.08 0.06	+15.0 to −15.0 Plano to −15.0	DW EW	Non pHEMA
Polysoft	67.5	8.3, 8.6, 8.9, 9.2	14.0	0.15	+15.0 to −15.0	DW or EW	Non pHEMA
Wohlk							
Hydroflex/M	38	7.1 to 9.1 in 0.1 steps	12.0, 12.5, 13.0, 13.5	0.10	+20.0 to −20.0	DW	pHEMA
Hydroflex/SD	38	7.6 to 8.8 in 0.4 steps	13.0, 13.5	0.08	+10.0 to −10.0	DW/ EW	pHEMA
		8.4 to 9.2 in 0.4 steps	14.5		+10.0 to +20.0		pHEMA
Weflex 55	55	8.1 to 9.0 in 0.3 steps	13.7	0.16	+10.0 to −20.0	DW	Non pHEMA
		8.4 to 9.3 in 0.3 steps	14.3	0.16	+10.0 to −20.0	DW	Non pHEMA
UNITED STATES OF AMERICA							
American Hydron							
Zero 6 (polymacon)	38	8.4, 8.7, 9.0	14.0	0.06	Plano to −10.0 in 0.25 steps	DW	pHEMA
Zero 4 (polymacon)	38	8.6	13.8	0.04	Plano to −8.50 in 0.25 steps	DW	pHEMA
Spincast (polymacon)	38	Aspheric	14.5	0.07	Plano to −8.00 in 0.25 steps	DW	pHEMA
Barnes-Hind Inc							
Hydrocurve II (bufilcon A)	45	8.6, 8.3 8.9	13.5 14.5	0.08 to 1.0	Plano to −12.0 +0.25 to	DW	pHEMA
		9.2, 9.5, 9.8, 10.1	15.5	0.08 to 1.0	+7.00 in 0.25 steps Plano to	DW	pHEMA
		9.5, 9.8	15.5		−20.0		
		9.2, 9.5, 9.8, 10.1	16.0	0.08 to 1.0	+0.25 to +7.00	DW	pHEMA
				0.08 to 1.0	in 0.25 steps Plano to −20.0 in 0.25 steps		
Softmate B (bufilcon A)	45	8.7, 9.0	14.3, 14.8	0.07 to 1.0	+7.00 to −12.00 in 0.25 steps	DW	pHEMA

Manufacturer/ Lens	Water %	BOZR (mm)	Diameter (mm)	CT at −3.00 DS	Powers (DS)	Wearing time	Material and remarks
Ciba Vision care							
Cibasoft (tefilcon A)	37.5	8.3, 8.6, 8.9	13.8	0.12	+6.00 to −10.00 in 0.25 steps	DW	pHEMA
		8.6, 8.9, 9.2	14.5	0.09 to 0.04	Plano to −10.0 in 0.25 steps		
Cibathin (tefilcon A)	37.5	8.6, 8.9	13.8	0.035	−1.00 to −6.00 in 0.25 steps	DW	pHEMA
Aosoft Minus (tetrafilcon A)	42.5		13.2	0.08 to 0.17	0.0 to −9.75		
Aosoft low plus (tetrafilcon A)	42.5		13.2	0.17 to 0.28	+0.25 to +6.50 in 0.25 steps	DW	pHEMA
Aosoft super thin (petrafilcon A)	42.5	8.2, 8.6	14.25	0.05 to 0.07	−0.25 to −7.75 in 0.25 steps	DW	pHEMA
Softcon (vifilcon A)	55	7.8, 8.1, 8.4, 8.7	14.0	0.10 to 0.64	−8.00 to +5.00 in 0.25 steps +5.00 to +18.0 in 0.50 steps	EW	pHEMA
		8.1, 8.4, 8.7	14.5		−8.0 to +5.00 in 0.25 steps, +5.0 to +18.0 in 0.50 steps		
Coopervision							
Standard Minus (tetrafilcon A)	42.5		13.2	0.10 to 0.18	Plano to −9.75 in 0.25 steps	DW	pHEMA
Superthin Minus (tetrafilcon A)	42.5		13.8	0.05 to 0.10	−0.25 to −20.00 in 0.25 steps	DW	pHEMA
Cooper Thin (polymacon)	38	8.4	14.0	0.06	−0.25 to −5.0 in 0.25 steps, −5.50 to −10.0 in 0.50 steps	DW	pHEMA
		8.6	14.5	0.06	−0.25 to −6.00 in 0.25 steps		
Super Thin Low Plus (tetrafilcon A)	42.5		13.8	0.11 to 0.39	Plano to +9.75 in 0.25 steps	DW	pHEMA
Permathin (tetrafilcon A)	42.5	8.4	13.8	0.035	Plano to −9.75 in 0.25 steps	DW	pHEMA
		8.9	14.4	0.035	Plano to 9.75 in 0.25 steps		
Metro Optics Inc							
Metrosoft II (polymacon)	38	8.3, 8.6, 8.9	13.5		+20.0 to −20.0	DW	pHEMA
Metro 55 (methafilcon A)	55	8.4, 8.7, 9.0	14.2		+20.0 to −20.0	DW	pHEMA

Manufacturer/ Lens	Water %	BOZR (mm)	Diameter (mm)	CT at −3.00 DS	Powers (DS)	Wearing time	Material and remarks
Syntex Ophthalmics							
CSI (crofilcon A)	38	8.0, 8.3, 8.6	13.8		−20.0 to +8.0	DW	Non pHEMA
Vistakon Inc							
HydroMarc spherical (etafilcon A)	43	8.15 to 9.05	14.0, 14.5		Plano to +10.0 +10.50 to +20.0	DW	Non pHEMA
Wesley Jessen							
Durasoft 2 (phemifilcon A)	38	8.3, 8.6, 9.0	14.5		+20.0 to −20.0	DW	pHEMA
Durasoft 3 (phemifilcon A)	55	8.3, 8.6, 9.0	14.5		+20.0 to −20.0	DW	pHEMA

Table A8.3 Examples of available Bausch and Lomb thin spuncast lenses

Lens series	Power range* (DS)	Diameter (mm)	Centre thickness (mm)
Sofspin	−0.25 to −12.00	14.00	0.05 to 0.09
U	−0.25 to −9.00	12.50	0.07
U3	−9.00 to +6.00	13.50	0.07 to 0.18
U4	−9.00 to +6.00	14.50	0.07 to 0.18
L3	−0.25 to −3.00	13.50	0.06
L4	−0.25 to −3.00	14.50	0.06
B3	−20.00 to +6.00	13.50	0.12 to 0.30
B4	−9.00 to +6.00	14.50	0.12 to 0.30
O3	−1.00 to −9.00	13.50	0.035
O4	−1.00 to −9.00	14.50	0.035

Lens powers from plano to ±5.00 D are in 0.25 steps, and from ±5.00 D to ±20.00 D in 0.50 D steps.

Table A8.4 Examples of available extended wear soft lenses

Manufacturer/Lens	Water %	Centre thickness (mm)	Diameter (mm)	BOZR (mm)	Powers (DS)	Material
UNITED KINGDOM						
Bausch and Lomb						
03/04	38	0.035 at −3.0 DS	03:13.5 04:14.5		0.25 to −5.0 in 0.25 steps, −5.50 and 6.00	pHEMA spuncast
B & L 70	70	Minus powers 0.14 Plus powers 0.16 to 0.25	14.3	8.4, 8.7, 9.0	Plano to −5.0 in 0.25 steps −5.50 and −6.60 +0.25 to +5.00 in 0.25 steps +5.5 and 6.0	Non pHEMA
B & L PW	79	0.49 to 0.79	14.4	8.1, 8.4, 8.7	All powers	Non pHEMA
Ciba Vision						
Weicon CE	60	0.09 at −3.0 DS	13.0, 13.8, 14.6	Flat and Steep	+20.0 to −20.0	Non pHEMA
Scanlens 75	71	0.12 at −4.0	13.3 14.0	7.9, 8.1, 8.3, 8.5 8.3, 8.5, 8.7, 8.9	+8.00 to −8.00 in 0.25 steps	Non pHEMA
		0.58 at +15.0	13.3 14.0	7.9, 8.1, 8.3, 8.5 8.1, 8.3, 8.5, 8.7	+8.50 to +20.0 in 0.50 steps	Non pHEMA
Contact Lenses Manufacturing						
PW	79	0.18 at −3.0 DS	13.0, 13.7, 14.4	7.5, 7.8, 8.1 8.4, 8.7		
Cooper Vision						
Permaflex 43		0.035 at −3.0 DS	14.4	8.4	Plano to −10.0	Non pHEMA lathe cut
Permaflex 74		0.14 at −3.0 DS	13.8	8.70 8.90	+5.0 to −10.0 Plano to −6.0	Non pHEMA Cast moulded
Permalens	71	0.10 to 0.43	13.5 14.0	7.4, 7.7, 8.0, 8.3 8.0, 8.3, 8.6	−0.25 to −5.0 in 0.25 steps −5.25 to 20.0 in 0.50 steps +0.25 to +5.0 in 0.25 steps +5.25 to +20.0 in 0.50 steps	Non pHEMA
Hydron (UK)						
H67	67%	0.15 for minus powers	14.0	8.0, 8.4, 8.8	Plano to ±10.0 in 0.25 steps ±10.0 to ±20.0 in 0.50 steps	Non pHEMA
Vistakon						
Acuvue Disposable	58	0.07	14.0	8.8	0.5 to 6.0 in 0.25 steps	Non pHEMA
Wohlk						
Geaflex 70	70	0.24 at −3.0 DS	13.4 14.2	7.8, 8.1, 8.4, 8.7 8.1, 8.4, 8.7, 9.0, 9.3	Plano to −20.0 Plano to +10.0 Plano to −20.0 Plano to +20.0 All in steps of 0.25	

Manufacturer/lens	Water %	Centre thickness (mm)	Diameter (mm)	BOZR (mm)	Powers (DS)	Material
UNITED STATES OF AMERICA						
American Hydron						
Hydron X70	70	0.14 to 0.17	14.3	8.4, 8.7, 8.9	Plano to −8.0	Non pHEMA
Barnes Hind						
Hydrocurve II	55	0.5 to 0.7	14.5	8.5, 8.8, 9.1	+7.0 to −12.0	Non pHEMA
Bausch and Lomb						
CW 79	79	0.5 to 0.7	14.4	8.1, 8.4, 8.7	+10.0 to +20.0	
70	70	0.14	14.3	8.4, 8.7, 9.0	+5.0 to −7.0	Non pHEMA
Ciba Vision Care						
CIBA 55	55	0.06 to 0.125	14.0	8.1, 8.4, 8.7	−0.5 to −6.0	Non pHEMA
Cooper Vision						
Permalens	71	0.10 to 0.43	13.5, 14.0, 14.5	8.0, 8.3, 8.6, 8.9	+20.0 to −10.0	Non pHEMA
Visiontech						
Sauflon PW	79	0.12 to 0.39	13.7, 14.4	7.5, 7.8, 8.1, 8.4, 8.7	Plano to +35.0	Non pHEMA
Vistakon						
Vistamarc	58	0.07	14.0, 14.5	8.0, 8.3, 8.6, 8.7	+7.0 to −9.0	Non pHEMA
Wesley Jessen						
Durasoft 3	55		13.5	8.2, 8.5	+20.0 to −20.0	Non pHEMA
			14.5	8.3, 8.6, 9.0		

Table A8.5 Examples of available toric soft contact lenses

Manufacturer/ Lens	Water %	Diameter (mm)	BOZR (mm)	Front (F) or Back (B)	Stabilization	Spherical powers (DS)	Cylinder powers (DC)	Axes
UNITED KINGDOM								
Bausch and Lomb								
Toric	45	14.0	8.3, 8.6	F	Prism	+4.0 to −6.0 in 0.25 steps	−1.25, −2.0	180° ± 20° 90° ± 20° in 10° steps
Ciba Vision								
Weicon TD Torisoft	38	14.5	8.6, 8.9, 9.2	F	Thin zones (slab off)	Plano to −7.0	−1.00, −1.75	180° ± 20° 90° ± 20° in 10° steps
Weicon T	38	15.0	8.2 to 9.6 in 0.2 steps	F	Thin zones (slab off)	+20.0 to −20.0	−1.0 to −4.0 in 0.25 steps	All
Hydron Europe								
Stock Toric	38	14.3	8.3 (moulded)	F	Prism and truncation	−1.0 to −6.0 in 0.25 steps	−0.75 to −2.0 in 0.25 steps	180° ± 20° 90° ± 20° in 10° steps
Rx Toric	38	13.0, 13.5, 14.0, 14.5, 15.0	7.9 to 8.9 in 0.1 steps	F	Prism and truncation	+20.0 to −20.0 in 0.25 steps	−0.50 to −6.0 in 0.25 steps	All
Hydron Z6T	38.6	14.0	8.4, 8.7, 9.0, 9.3		Prism 1.00D	Plano to ±10.0 in 0.25 steps, ±10.0 to ±20.0 in 0.50 steps	−0.50 to −6.0 in 0.25 steps	0° to 180°

Manufacturer/ lens	Water %	Diameter (mm)	BOZR (mm)	Front (F) or Back (B)	Stabilization	Spherical powers (DS)	Cylinder powers (DC)	Axes
Lunelle								
Rx Toric	70	14.3	8.3, 8.6, 8.9	F	2 raised zones at 3 & 9 o'clock	+8.0 to −8.0	−0.5 to −2.5 in 0.25 steps	All
		15.0	8.7, 8.9, 9.1	F		+20.0 to −20.0	−0.50 to −6.00 in 0.25 steps	
Pilkington Barnes Hind								
Hydrocurve II	45	13.5	8.6	B	Prism	+3.0 to −6.25 in 0.25 steps	−1.25 to −2.0	180° ± 25° 90° ± 25° in 5° steps
		14.5	8.9	B		+3.00 to −8.0 in 0.25 steps	−1.25 to −2.0	All in 5° steps
	55	14.5	8.8	B	Prism	+4.0 to −8.0 in 0.25 steps	−0.75, −1.25 and −2.0	All in 5° steps
			8.5	B	Prism	+3.0 to −8.0 in 0.25 steps	−1.25	180° ± 25° 90° ± 25° in 5° steps
Vistakon								
Hydromarc Toric	58	14.5	8.6	F	Prism with thin zone (slab off)	+4.0 to −5.0 in 0.25 steps	−0.75 to −2.5 in 0.25 steps	180° ± 20° 90° ± 20° in 5° steps
Wohlk								
TS	38	14.0, 15.0	8.1 to 10.0 in 0.1 steps	B	Prism and truncation	+20.0 to −20.0 in 0.25 steps	−0.50 to −6.0 in 0.5 steps	All
MT	38	12.0, 12.5, 13.0, 13.5	7.1 to 9.00 in 0.1 steps	B	Prism	+20.0 to −20.0 in 0.25 steps	−0.50 to −6.0 in 0.5 steps	All
AT	38	12.5, 13.0, 13.5	7.3 to 9.0 in 0.1 steps	F	Prism	As above	As above	All
UNITED STATES OF AMERICA								
American Hydron								
Zero T	38	14.5	8.3	B	Prism and truncations	−1.0 to −4.0 in 0.25 steps	0.75 to −2.00 in 0.25 steps	180° ± 20° 90° ± 20° in 10° steps
Custom Toric	38	13.5, 14.5	7.2 to 9.2 in 0.1 steps	B	Prism and truncation	Plano to +9.0 in 0.25 steps, +9.50 to +20.0 in 0.50 steps	−0.50 to −6.5	All
Barnes Hind Same as for UK above								
Bausch and Lomb Same as for UK above								
Ciba Vision Same as for UK above (Weicon TD Torisoft)								
Vistakon								
Hydromarc minus toric	43	14.5	8.45, 8.75, 9.05	F	Prism and slab off	Plano to −5.0 in 0.25 steps	−0.75 to −2.0 in 0.25 steps	180: ± 20° 90° ± 20° in 5° steps
Hydromarc	43	14.5	8.75, 9.05			+0.25 to +5.0 in 0.25 steps		
Wesley Jessen								
Durasoft TT	38	13.5	7.8, 8.3, 8.6, 9.0	F	Prism and truncation	+20.0 to −20.0 in 0.25 steps	−0.75 to 4.0 in 0.25 steps, −4.0 to −8.0 in 0.50 steps	180° ± 20° 90° ± 20° in 5° steps
Durasoft 2 Toric	38	13.5	8.2, 8.5	F	Prism and truncation	+20.0 to −20.0 in 0.25 steps	−0.75 to −3.0 in 0.25 steps	180° ± 20° 90° ± 20° in 5° steps
		14.5	8.3, 8.6	F				
Durasoft 3 Toric	55	14.5	8.3, 8.6	F	Prism and truncation	+4.0 to −8.0	−0.75 to −2.0 in 0.25 steps	180° ± 30° 90° ± 30° in 5° steps

Table A8.6 Examples of available soft and rigid lenses to correct presbyopia

SOFT LENSES

Manufacturer/ Lens	Water %	Diameter (mm)	BOZR (mm)	Distance power in dioptres	Near add in dioptres	Distance diameter (mm)	Design
Alges						Near diameter	
Bifocal	45	14.0	8.6, 8.9	+4.0 to −4.0 in 0.25 steps, +4.5 to +6.0 and −4.5 to 6.0 in 0.50 steps	2.0, 2.5, 3.0, 3.5	2.12, 2.35, 2.55, 3.0, 3.5	Concentric near central
Bausch and Lomb							
PA1	38	13.5	N/A spuncast	+5.0 to −5.0 in 0.25 steps, +5.5 and +6.0	Progressive to +2.0	N/A	Aspheric back curve concentric – distance
Crescent bifocal	45	14.0	8.6, 8.9	−0.25 to −6.0 in 0.25 steps	+1.5 +2.0		Crescent segment Prism and truncation
		13.5	8.6, 8.9	Plano to +6.0 in 0.25 steps	+2.5		
Ciba Vision							
Weicon 38E Bisoft	38	13.0, 13.8		+7.0 to −7.0 in 0.25 steps	1.5 to 3.0	3.2, 3.8	Concentric distance central
Nissel							
PS45 Presbyopic soft lens	38	14	8.7	−2.00 to +4.00	+2.00	About 4	Multifocal design
Pilkington Barnes Hind							
Hydrocurve II Bifocal	45	14.8	9.0	+4.0 to −6.0 in 0.25 steps	Progressive to +1.5	4	Aspheric back curve concentric distance central
Wesley Jessen							
Durasoft 2 bifocal (phemifilcon A)	38	13.5	8.5	+4.5 to −4.5	+1.0 to +2.75 in 0.25 steps		Crescent segment Prism and truncation

RIGID LENSES

Manufacturer/ Lens	Material	Dk at 35°C (mm)	Total diameter (mm)	BOZR (mm)	Distance power in dioptres	Near add in dioptres	Design
Ciba Vision Titmus							
Selecon bifocal	PMMA	NIL	9.5, 10.0	7.2 to 8.65 in 0.05 steps	+20.0 to −20.0	+1.0 to +3.0 in 0.25 steps	Crescent segment Prism and truncation
Pilkington							
Diffrax	Polycon II Silicone + Methylmeth-acrylate	12	9.5	7.0 to 8.4 in 0.1 steps	+6.0 to −6.0 in 0.25 steps	+1.0 to +3.0 in 0.5 steps	Hologram diameter 5mm

Table A8.7 Basic PMMA trial lenses for keratoconus

BOZR	BOZD	First BPZR	First BPZD	Second BBZR	Total diameter	Power (DS)
7.20	7.0	8.20	7.80	10.20	8.40	− 4.00
7.00	7.0	8.00	7.80	10.00	8.40	− 6.00
6.80	7.0	7.80	7.80	9.80	8.40	− 8.00
6.60	7.0	7.60	7.80	9.60	8.40	− 8.00
6.40	7.0	7.40	7.80	9.40	8.40	− 8.00
6.20	7.0	7.20	7.80	9.20	8.40	−10.00
6.00	7.0	7.00	7.80	9.00	8.40	−12.00
5.80	7.0	6.80	7.80	8.80	8.40	−14.00
5.60	7.0	6.60	7.80	8.60	8.40	−16.00
5.40	7.0	6.40	7.80	8.40	8.40	−18.00

Table A8.8 Ciba Vision Persecon E. Keratoconus lenses

BOZR in steps of 0.1 mm

from	to	Powers (DS)	TD	FOZD
5.90	7.60		9.30	8.0
6.00	7.70	±20.00	9.80	8.5

Trial lens powers	
7.70–7.30	− 2.50 DS
7.20–6.80	− 5.00 DS
6.70–6.30	− 7.50 DS
6.20–5.90	−10.00 DS

Initial trial lens

Flattest K reading	Add in mm to flattest K reading
7.60–6.80	Nil
6.80–6.60	0.50 mm
6.0 −5.5	0.80 mm
5.00 and steeper	1.00 mm

Table A8.9 Examples of available soft translucent tinted contact lenses

Manufacturer/ Lens	Material	Tints	Water %	BOZR (mm)	Iris diameter (mm)	Pupil diameter (mm)	TD (mm)	Powers in 0.25 DS
Bausch and Lomb Natural tint	pHEMA spuncast	Blue, aqua, green, yellow, brown	38		11.0		U3 13.5 (0.07) U4 14.5 (0.07) B3 13.5 (0.12)	−0.25 to −5.0 in 0.25 steps and −5.5 and 6.0
Ciba Vision Ellipticolours	pHEMA lathe cut	Amber, aqua, blue, green, 10 and 20% absorption	38	Flat Steep	TD		13.0, 13.8, 14.6	+20.0 to −20.0
Cooper Vision Permaflex colour collection	CP, MMA and VP	Violet, blue, skyblue, golden, spring green, turquoise	74	8.7	11.2	5.0	14.4	Plano to −6.0 in 0.25 steps
Hydron UK Soft Tints		Aqua, emerald, smokey quartz In 10% or 20%	38	8.7	11.5	4.5	see below	Z6 and Mini +20.0 to −20.0

Available in Zero 6, Mini, Z4 and Spincast (Table A8.2)

Manufacturer/ Lens	Material	Tints	Water %	BOZR (mm)	Iris diameter (mm)	Pupil diameter (mm)	TD (mm)	Powers in 0.25 DS
Igel International								
Hi tint CD	pHEMA	Sapphire blue	38	8.5, 8.7, 8.9		2.0 to 6.0 in 1mm steps in	14.0	+20.0 to −20.0
Hi tint 67	Terpolymer of Vp	Aqua, emerald, topaz, amber	67	8.3, 8.7, 9.1	10.0 to 12.0 in 0.50 steps	clear and 3.0 to 9.0 with black pupil	14.0	+20.0 to −20.0
Hi tint 77	Terpolymer of Vp	Smokey brown	76.5	8.4, 8.8, 9.2			14.0	+10.0 to −10.0
Nissel								
Hypa II	pHEMA	Blue, aqua-marine, green, yellow, brown	37	8.7	10.0		14.0	Plano to −10.0 in 0.25 steps and Plano to +10.0 in 0.50 steps
Pilkington Barnes Hind								
Softmate	pHEMA/DDA/ MMA and	Sapphire blue, aquamarine,	45	9.0	11.0	4	14.8	Plano to −8.0
	TMPTMA	emerald green, topaz	55	9.0	10.0	4	14.8	+6.0 to −8.0
Wohlk								
Hydroflex Colour	pHEMA	3 grey, 2 blue, 2 brown and green	38	8.3 to 9.90 in 0.1 steps	A 11.0 B as TD C as TD D 10.0, 11.5	4 3.0, 4.0, 5.0, 6.0	13.0, 13.5 12.0, 12.5, 13.0, 13.5 12.0, 12.5, 13.0, 13.5	+20.0 to −20.0 in 0.25 steps
Weflex 55	Poly-acyl MA	Green, turquoise, blue, brown	55	8.1, 8.4, 8.7, 9.0	11.0	4	13.7	+20.0 to −20.0 with clear pupil or solid tint
	NVP		55	8.4, 8.7, 9.0, 9.3	11.5	4	14.3	

Table A8.10 Examples of available soft opaque tinted contact lenses

Manufacturer/ Lens	Material	Tints	Water %	BOZR (mm)	Iris diameter (mm)	Pupil diameter (mm)	TD (mm)	Powers in 0.25 DS steps
Contact Lenses Manufacturing Aquarius		Base, radial, corona patterns in light, medium or dark blue, green, aqua, yellow	77 79	All	12.0, 12.5, 13.0	3.4, 4.5	13.0 13.7 14.4	All
Coopervision Mystique	Permaflex	Sapphire, dark, crystal and light blue; willow, light jade and dark green	38	8.7	12.0	4.2, 4.7	14.2	Plano to −6.0 in 0.25 steps
Hydron Soft colour		Aqua, sapphire, emerald, smokey, quartz, amber			11.5	4.5	see below	Z6 and Mini +20.0 to −20.0
		Available in Zero 6, Mini, Z4 and Spincast (Table A8.2)						
Igel International	Terpolymer of VP		67 77	8.3, 8.7, 9.1 8.4, 8.8, 9.2	10.0, 10.5, 11.0, 11.50, 12.0	3.0, 3.5, 4.0, 4.5, 5.0, 5.5, 6.0, 7.0, 8.0 and 9.0 in designs A and D 2.0, 3.0, 4.0, 5.0 and 6.0 in design C	14.0	+20.0 to −20.0 +10.0 to −10.0 both in 0.25 steps
		A B C D						
Vistakon UV Bloc	Etafilcon A	UV Filter	58	8.4, 8.7, 8.8			14.0 14.0 14.5	+4.0 to −6.0

Table A8.11 Examples of printed and hand painted cosmetic lenses

Manufacturer/Lens	Water %	BOZR (mm)	TD (mm)	Iris diameter (mm)	Pupil diameter (mm)	Colours	Powers (DS)
Ciba Vision							
Weicon Iris print soft lens	38	8.4 to 9.6 in 0.2 steps	15.0	11.5	4.5 clear or black	Green, grey, blue	+20.0 to −20.0 in 0.25 steps
Weicon Iris hand painted soft lens	38	8.4 to 9.6 in 0.2 steps	15.0	11.5 or to order	4.5 or to order, clear or black	According to sample	As above
Nissel							
Painted PMMA lens		to order	11.5	to order	to order	According to sample	+20.0 to −20.0 in 0.25 steps

Table A8.12 Examples of available therapeutic soft contact lenses in plano power

Manufacturer	Name	Water %	Centre thickness	BOZR (mm)	Diameter (mm)
Bausch and Lomb	O4	38.6	0.06	Spuncast	14.5
Bausch and Lomb	B4	38.6	0.12	Spuncast	14.5
Hydron Europe	O4	38.6	0.04	8.6	13.8
Pilkington Contact Lenses	CSIT	38.5	0.035	8.0, 8.3, 8.6 8.6, 8.9, 9.35	13.8 14.8
Ciba Vision (USA)	Softcon	55	0.10	8.10, 8.4, 8.7 8.7	14.0 14.5
Pilkington/Barnes Hind	Hydrocurve II	55	0.06	9.1, 9.8	14.0 16.0
Wohlk	Bandage Hydroflex 72	72	0.15	8.2, 8.5, 8.8, 9.1, 9.4	14.5
Cooper Vision	Permalens	71	0.21	7.7, 8.0, 8.3, 8.6	13.5 14.2
Ciba Vision	Scanlens	75	0.12	8.5	14.0 15.0
Contact Lens Manufacturing (UK)	Sauflon PW	79	0.45	8.4, 8.7	15.5
Vision Tech (USA)	Sauflon PW	79	0.45	8.1, 8.4, 8.7	14.4

Bibliography

AQUAVELLA, J.V. and RAO, G.N. (eds) (1987) *Contact Lenses*, J.B. Lippincott, Philadelphia and London

COHEN, E.J. (ed.) (1986) Contact lenses and external disease. *International Ophthalmology Clinics*, **26** (1), Little, Brown and Company, Boston

DABEZIES, O.H. (ed.) (1984) *Contact Lenses. The Contact Lens Association of Ophthmologists guide to basic science and clinical practice* (2 volumes and 3 updates), Grune and Stratton, New York and London

GRAYSON, M.G. (1983) *Diseases of the Cornea*, 2nd edn, C.V. Mosby, St. Louis, Toronto, and London

HALES, R.H. (1982) *Contact Lenses*, 2nd edn, Williams and Wilkins, Baltimore and London

LEE, J.R. (1986) *Contact Lens Handbook*, W.B. Saunders, Philadelphia and London

LEIBOWITZ, H.M. (ed.) (1984) *Cornea Disorders*, W.B. Saunders, Philadelphia and London

MILLER, D. and WHITE, P.F. (eds) (1981) Complications of contact lenses. *International Ophthalmology Clinics*, **21** (2), Little, Brown and Company, Boston

OLSON, R.J. (1984) Common corneal problems. *International Ophthalmology Clinics*, **24** (2), Little, Brown and Company, Boston

RUBEN, M. (ed.) (1975) *Contact Lens Practice*, Bailliere Tindall, London

RUBEN, M. (ed.) (1978) *Soft Contact Lenses*, Bailliere Tindall, London

RUBEN, M. (1982) *A Colour Atlas of Contact Lenses*, Wolfe Medical Publications, London

SMOLIN, G. and THOFT, R.A. (eds) (1987) *The Cornea*, 2nd edn, Little, Brown and Company, Boston and Toronto

STIEN, A.S. and SLATT, B.J. (1984) *Fitting Guide for Rigid and Soft Contact Lenses*, 2nd edn, C.V. Mosby, St. Louis and Toronto

STENSON, S.M. (ed.) (1987) *Contact Lenses*, Appleton and Lange, Norwalk, Connecticut

STONE, J. and PHILLIPS, A.J. (eds) (1980) *Contact Lenses*, 2nd edn, Butterworths, London and Boston

Index